The First 16
Secrets of CHI

To DAME KAREN

HEALTH IS WEALTH

健身 就是 財富

Bond

The First 16 Secrets of CHI

Feng Shui for the Human Body

Luk Chun Bond
Chi Kung Master

text prepared by
U'i and Steven Goldsberry

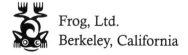
Frog, Ltd.
Berkeley, California

Published by Frog, Ltd.

Frog, Ltd. books are distributed by
North Atlantic Books
P.O. Box 12327
Berkeley, California 94712

Cover photograph by
Book design by Paula Morrison

Printed in the United States of America

North Atlantic Books' publications are available through most bookstores. For further information, call 800-337-2665 or visit our website at www.northatlanticbooks.com.

Substantial discounts on bulk quantities are available to corporations, professional associations, and other organizations. For details and discount information, contact our special sales department.

Library of Congress Cataloging-in-Publication Data
Chun Bond, Luk.
    The first sixteen secrets of chi : feng shui for the human body / by Luk Chun Bond, with U'i and Steven Goldsberry.
        p. cm.
    ISBN 1-58394-052-9 (alk. paper)
    1. Qi gong. 2. Feng shui. 3. Physical fitness. 4. Longevity.
    5. Health. I. Title.
RA781.8 .C484 2001
613.7—dc21
                                                            2001033426

2 3 4 5 6 7 8 9 / 05 04 03 02

Dedication

This book is dedicated to my father, Luk Man Niu, who passed the knowledge of this precious, ancient art of healing on to me, and to my mother, Chau Kwai Fan, whose dying wish was that I remain steadfast in perpetuating this legacy.

Disclaimer

Those under treatment by a physician should continue their medical care and are advised to seek their physician's permission before proceeding with any exercise program or changes in diet.

Table of Contents

How to Use This Book

For centuries, Buddhist and Taoist monks of China have studied ways to master the human body—cure its ills, control the mind, and increase longevity.

With encouragement and support from many ruling dynasties, the Chinese practice of traditional holistic healing developed into the art form described in the *I Ching* as t'ai chi.

T'ai chi has been introduced to Western cultures as a choreographed series of slow, methodical movements performed in meditative silence. In fact, it is much more than this.

The 108 movements currently taught are just a tiny part of the whole of t'ai chi. The term "t'ai chi" describes a combination of disciplines:

1. T'ai Chi Ch'uan—the slow, dance-like movements widely practiced in China, and taught in classes around the United States.

2. External Chi Kung—the martial art form known as kung fu, used for self-defense.

3. Internal Chi Kung, or breathing power therapy—used for protection and healing.

4. Feng shui—the study of the movement of the chi life force (bio-magnetic fields) of the earth and sky. The magnetic fields around certain areas influence the electrical system, better known as the central nervous system, of the human body.

I teach the Cheung San Fung method, a practical combination of the four main disciplines of t'ai chi. Originally developed during the Sung Dynasty by the Taoist monk Cheung San Fung, this proven style of self-healing is still practiced in urban parks and rural fields throughout the great country of China. It has often been referred to as the "never changing style" of t'ai chi, and is famous for its nearly magical ability to assist the human immune system in creating a healthier, stronger body and mind.

I have taught classes all over the world—from London and Paris to the islands of Hawai'i. I have witnessed the Cheung San Fung method help many people who suffer from back pain, diabetes, Alzheimer's disease, asthma, arthritis, weight disorders, hypertension, Parkinson's disease, and the ravages of daily stress. Students arrive at class in Jaguars and Mercedes and Fords, on wheelchairs, in city buses, and on foot, and they tell me of their battles with strokes and heart attacks.

My classes are free, and my only request is that my students take the exercises I teach and do them faithfully for at least thirty minutes each day. Some of the weaker pupils break their workouts into tiny segments of time from ten 3-minute sessions to three 10-minute sessions, daily. It doesn't matter where they start. It's just important that they begin, and that 30 minutes a day is focused on their healing and overall health.

The ancient discipline of t'ai chi incorporates the utilization of the vital life force that the Chinese call "chi."

Chi is the energy that heals us, emanates from us, and binds us together in the matrix of life on this planet. It is created by all living things, and flows freely throughout our world, and through us.

To describe chi movement in the landscapes of our physical environment, the Chinese use the term "feng shui." From my father's instruction, my experiences traveling, and in teaching my classes, I've developed a keen understanding of the profound similarities in the way chi moves through a landscape and the way it moves through the human body. I use this connection to help my students understand that as they bring chi into their systems, it flows through meridians and channels that feed and nourish vital organs, tissues, muscles, glands, and bones, and that the positioning of the body—which body parts are tightened, stretched, and elongated—is important to chi flow. Just as the location of a window, door, chair, or plant in a house either blocks or accelerates chi movement, the postures we practice will enhance energy flow to areas in need of rejuvenation. And our location when we exercise has profound influence on our success. This is feng shui for the human body.

With this in mind, I've compiled a very simple course of breathing techniques, physical exercises, and meditations that are rooted in the high-mountain monasteries of the Buddhist and Taoist monks, where the secrets of longevity have been cloistered for centuries. I've adapted them slightly to fit the lifestyle of the 21st century. The basic concepts of feng shui are an integral part of these techniques for health and long life.

This book is a way for me to pass on the knowledge handed down from the monks of a Taoist monastery to my grandfather, to my father, and to me. To anyone looking for relief from emotional, physical, and spiritual distress, and for those who want a healthier and happier life, the secrets of chi revealed in these pages provide a very easy program to follow.

To get the most from these lessons, read each chapter through first, then reread key elements as you work on your exercises, making sure that your location and techniques are correct.

The exercises are prescriptive, which means that each one will help to cure certain ailments as well as strengthen your immune system. In life, at any moment, we are either spiraling down toward disease or spiraling up toward health. Every time you perform one of these exercises you are spiraling up, getting better and stronger.

Take this knowledge and make it your own. Just 30 minutes a day will fill you with the healthy vigor of youth.

Good luck, prosperity, and good health.

Masters of the Secret Chi

Before I was born, my father moved our family from the province of Canton to a farm on a steep hillside on the outskirts of Lei Yue Mun village, near Hong Kong. From our fields I watched the sampans and junks float in and out of the narrow channel, and at night across the waters of Victoria Harbor we could see the lights of the great city.

For a time my father worked in Hong Kong, but he also worked with our family on the farm. In the evenings after our chores were done, he often told us stories. My favorites were the tales of my grandfather. He became a character of myth to me, a legend spoken of with reverence and honor. And although I never met him, for he passed away soon after I was born, my grandfather gave me my purpose, and the teachings I needed to fulfill my life's mission.

My only recollections of my grandfather are these stories, which make a sort of collective family memory shared by all my father's children.

Grandfather's name was Luk Hock Choun, which means crane and pine, both symbols of longevity and strength. When I think of his name I see a great green pine tree alone in a field, and beneath its boughs a crane standing on one strong leg, its white feathers shining.

Grandfather worked as an herbal doctor in the village of Wai Chow, tending to the physical, emotional, and spiritual well-being of the people there. His chi was strong and clear, and the villagers could sense its power just by looking at him.

Many years before my father was born, Luk Hock Choun had

journeyed to the Taoist monastery on the hilltop near his home village to learn t'ai chi and its healing component, chi kung. He met
two Supreme Monk disciples there, Zi Man and Chi Yat, who recognized Grandfather's gift for healing. They took him in and became
his sifu, his honorable teachers. Zi Man always carried a heavy
wooden staff made of solid teak, a very spiritual stick. He used it as
a tool to train his students in the peaceful art of mastering the vital
essence, chi. On very rare occasions, though, he used the staff to
defend himself when attacked by bandits on the remote trails and
paths that led to and from the monastery.

Over time, Zi Man let Grandfather practice using the staff. At
first it seemed too heavy, difficult to lift, and almost impossible to
wield. In one practice session Zi Man, a very old man, held the tip of
the 8-foot long stick between his thumb and forefinger, and sliced it
through the air like a sword. "Now you try," he said. "You must push
your chi through your fingers and into the staff. Make it part of your
body. Make it part of your energy." Grandfather held the staff as he
was told, but could not lift it.

One day, Zi Man extended his arm, holding the staff with his fingers, and said, "Luk Hock Choun, hold the staff in the middle."
Grandfather grabbed the shaft with two hands wrapped tightly around
the center. "Bend your elbows slightly. Extend. Hold the staff at arm's
length. Practice. Breathe. Bring the chi through your arms and into
the stick." Then Zi Man walked away, leaving Luk Hock Choun
alone in the monastery garden. Grandfather had a strong will, and a
most powerful desire to learn. He did as he was instructed. He held
the staff until his arms, shoulders, and neck ached. Each moment
the staff became heavier. Grandfather tried concentrating on his
breathing technique, but the growing pain in his muscles clouded his
mind. When Zi Man returned, he found Luk Hock Choun in a heap
on the rough tile floor, arms hugging his shoulders, forehead pressed
against the ground.

"The chi inside you is strong," Zi Man said, as he helped Luk
Hock Choun to his feet. "You will learn to control it with your breathing. The chi will make the staff light, like a tree trunk lifted by a great

monsoon wind." Zi Man handed Grandfather a 3-foot-long fig branch. "Hold it between your fingers."

Grandfather obeyed his sifu. The branch, although light as a leaf, caused a pain to surge through his arms. The muscles were still tender from his ordeal with the staff.

"Inhale the chi," Zi Man said. "Hold it in your dan tien." The master pointed to Grandfather's lower abdomen. "Now bring it up and push the chi through your arms. Breathe. Relax your shoulders. Let the chi lift everything. Close your eyes. The chi wants to help you. Let it lift the branch."

Grandfather concentrated. With his eyes closed, the branch disappeared. He felt his arms rise in one light, smooth movement. There was no effort. He opened his eyes and the pain returned. His arms dropped.

Master Zi Man shook his head. "You would do better if you were blind, I think. Come tomorrow. You can try again."

Grandfather returned early the next morning and did the chores the monks required their students to perform before training. When it was time, he went to the garden. Zi Man stood in the shade of a willow, his staff on the ground at his feet. A slight breeze rustled the long willow branches. "Come," Zi Man whispered. "This spot is strong with chi. It will help you in your lesson today."

Grandfather stood next to his sifu, in the pale green light beneath the willow. "Raise the staff," Zi Man commanded.

"Sifu, my whole body is sore," Grandfather complained. "I could barely lift the mop bucket to do my chores."

"You must learn to use the chi in every part of your life. It will make all of your chores effortless. Now, pick up the staff."

Grandfather bent over and grabbed the staff in the center. "Good," Zi Man said. "Close your eyes and let the chi lift it as it did the branch."

Grandfather struggled. "Move the chi," Zi Man commanded. "Move it through your body. It will join with the chi in the staff. Feel the heat rise from your abdomen, your dan tein, up your spine, through your shoulders, to your hands, and into the staff."

Grandfather felt it, and the staff became light, like lifting a finger. "Now, slowly move your hand down the staff to the end closest to you." Zi Man spoke in a whisper as he backed away from his student, his voice growing faint, blending with the murmurings of the willow. "Work your way to the very end. Let the chi guide your hand as you guide the staff."

For a long time, Grandfather held the heavy stick out in front of him, moving his hands in tiny increments until he reached the end. The staff extended at full length before him. "I did it, Sifu," he said. "Look." He opened his eyes, and turned, but the old master was gone, and the staff fell to the ground. That was the end of his second lesson.

Grandfather worked with the staff every day. Zi Man eventually stopped coming to the garden. Grandfather would arrive to find the staff lying in the grass beneath the willow.

One day, Grandfather arrived at the tree and saw Zi Man sitting cross-legged in meditation, the staff stretched out before him. Grandfather sat opposite the old master. With his eyes still closed, Zi Man said, "Pick up the staff with your fingers, and hand it to me." Grandfather sat down and closed his eyes, then reached for the tip of the stick, and held it out to the old man. Zi Man didn't move. "Raise it over your head," he said. Grandfather did as he was told. "Open your eyes and watch your actions." Again, Grandfather obeyed without effort.

"Good," said the old man. "You have learned to control and direct your chi. Take the staff. It is yours. It will serve you well."

Grandfather was surprised. "I need to learn more. I want to learn everything."

"That is everything," the old man said. "When you can move the chi through your body and connect with the outside world, you have mastered all I can teach you. The rest you will learn as the world sends you challenges."

Years later, Luk Hock Choun became a master, and then a double master, and finally a triple master. The staff became the symbol of Grandfather's training, like a magic wand that carried his knowledge in the dense fibers of the wood.

Luk Hock Choun taught his son, my father Luk Man Niu, the lessons of the monks, and when my father had successfully completed the training, the staff was handed down to him.

My father's name, Luk Man Niu, means "man who can live 60,000 years." He is now approaching age 99, and is strong and full of life. People say he looks 60. His students travel miles to learn from him the lessons of the Taoist monks.

As a young man (this was many years before I was born) Luk Man Niu worked for a printer in Hong Kong. When the Japanese army moved into the city during World War II, his life drastically changed. There was much lawlessness with the Japanese occupation. At night, thieves and bandits would descend upon our village, and steal pigs and chickens, bushels of stored rice and vegetables, anything they could carry.

Every evening my father came home on the barge that ferried workers from Hong Kong Island. The water near the shore was very shallow. A muddy shoal rose from the deep harbor channel along the coastline. When the barge neared the shore, crewmen heaved a one-foot-wide plank onto the pier for the passengers to disembark. The wood wobbled and bounced as men, women, and children, some carrying heavy packages, carefully walked single-file to the dock. It was common on rough days, when the wind flew wildly and the sea rocked the barge, for passengers to lose their footing and tumble into the cold, murky water. My father always said that balance and patience were the keys to having a dry trip home.

One day, the clouds rolled in thick and gray in the early afternoon, and the wind, chilled from miles of travel over the open ocean, whipped the inlet into froth-tipped waves. Father boarded the barge. He sat with a group of his friends, villagers and neighbors, and they talked about leaving their families each day, and their fear that the bandits would come early, before they got home to protect their farms. Our farm was high on the hill; a single dirt path was the only way in or out. My father knew that his young family was safe. So he listened to his friends' stories of terror, but did not share their dread. Until this time, he had kept his t'ai chi training a secret, not wanting to call attention to himself. He has always been an extremely humble man. But things in the village seemed to be getting much worse. To avoid harm, some families started the practice of leaving food from their fields on their doorsteps for the robbers, and took jobs in the city to compensate for the income loss. The robbers began expecting this and punished others for not making the same offerings. One angry woman looked over at my father and shook her finger. "Luk Man Niu!" she snarled. "Your wife, she sits on your mountain. You think she's safe? You think no bandit will bother her?" The woman stood up and staggered through the listing of the barge toward my father. "One day you will see, Luk Man Niu. They will visit your home while you are away. And there will be no food for them on your doorstep. You have heard what they do. Your wife, she is young. Your children are young. One day you will see."

The other people in the group told her to sit. The barge was tossing in the wind and waves. Father knew what he would do if the bandits dared attack his home. He slept each night with Grandfather's staff on the floor beside the sleeping mats. His training with Grandfather had been completed. He too had been made a double master. He would protect his family, and his farm.

According to the story, that night of the day the angry woman spoke her warning, my father was sleeping in his house with his family, and over the howling of the wind he heard his dogs bark, then yelp like someone had hit them. It was very dark. Black clouds blocked the small light of a slivered moon. Father rose slowly from his mats, and shook my mother. "Gather the children in the loft upstairs," he said. "Keep them quiet. I'll be back soon."

My mother did as she was told. She grabbed her little babies, bundled them in blankets, and hushed them back to sleep in the loft. She heard my father open the front door, then close it again. There was no other sound outside but the wind and the dogs.

Then, in the calm just before she fell asleep, Mother heard in the distance men's voices, angry voices, yelling. She sat up, away from the soft breathing of her children, and listened hard. There were sounds of wood hitting wood, of men shouting, and guttural screams of pain. Mother slumped back with her little ones, pulled the blankets over all of them, and waited.

She said it seemed like many hours before she heard the door creak open, and my father walk in and lean against the entry wall. She gently rose from her nest, and went to him.

He was bleeding, but nothing serious. "Are you all right?" she asked. She led him to a chair in the middle of the living room. "What happened? Was it the bandits?" She had so many questions. Father asked for hot tea, a special blend, a healing tea from the province of Canton.

Mother returned, carrying a steaming cup and a damp cloth. "How many were there?" she asked. She wiped away the blood from a forehead cut.

"I didn't count," Father said.

"Five? Ten? Give me a guess," she said. "The women at the market say that the bandits always travel in packs of five or more."

"I don't know," Father said. "Maybe ten. Maybe."

"Where are they now?" she asked.

"Let's return to bed. I'm not going to work tomorrow. I'm going to find their homes, and settle this. I will not live this way."

Father woke early, and went to the dock. He talked to some of the villagers as they waited for the barge, and asked one man to tell his boss he would not be at work. "You are really going to fight them?" a merchant asked. "I would like to see that."

Another man said, "I want your farm if you don't come back."

The angry woman from the barge the day before said, "What if they get upset at all of us? They could destroy the village. You are a very selfish man, Luk Man Niu. Foolish and selfish."

At that moment, the barge plank slapped onto the dock. "Good luck, Luk Man Niu," they all said, and they started their bobbing trek over the plank to the barge.

It took two days for father to locate the bandits' camp at the top of Devil's Hill. Using his staff as a walking stick, he climbed the narrow path that led to the hill's summit. Halfway up the hill, he was joined by four men from the village. "We've come to help," they said. "We're tired of living in fear."

The men finished the climb together.

Father and his band surveyed the camp from behind a clump of bushes. "How many are there?" one man asked. "It looks like between 60 and 80 men."

"That's what it looks like to me," another said. "Can we really do this?"

My father stood with his eyes closed, breathing in a way that made his abdomen move, but not his shoulders, the dan tien breathing. The other men watched. "Luk Man Niu," one said. "Are you all right?"

"Yes," Father said. "I am fine. I will enter first, and begin the fight alone. You may join in when you feel it's time." Then Father walked into the camp.

I've heard this story from my father, my mother, and many of the older men in the village, and each time it's told, the story is the same. Father walked into the camp, confronted the first men he saw, and started fighting. Using Grandfather's staff, he fought off over 60 bandits, while his four village friends took care of the other 20. When it was all over, Father returned home.

He'd suffered what seemed to be mild injury, a few cuts here and there, but he left the village and went to the mountain to heal himself. He told me many years later, while I was training to be a t'ai chi master, that he felt his meridians were hurt. He needed a strong dose of chi kung to heal the damage.

Grandfather heard of this battle, and sent a letter to my father asking him to come to Canton. When Father returned, he had been elevated to triple master.

Things were never the same in the village. The people stopped leaving their doorstep offerings. There were no reprisals. The bandits never raided again. It was said that they simply disappeared. One of our farmers hiked up Devil's Hill and found the campsite deserted, the livestock gone.

Many of the village men and their sons wanted my father to train them to do what he could do. So, in the years that followed, Father ran a t'ai chi school in the village, and held classes on days he wasn't in Hong Kong at the printing company. T'ai chi training became an integral part of our family life, and like the rest of my eleven brothers and sisters, I began my training at the age of six.

In the Luk family, if you could walk, you could work. There were so many chores. Days began at dawn, when the roosters crowed at the purple sky. Our schedule was breakfast, then chores, then school, then more chores.

Father hired a man to supervise his children in how to feed and care for the pigs, chickens, ducks, geese, pigeons, dogs, and fish; another man to supervise the tending of the vegetable garden; and a third man to handle the repairs on the farm.

Our chores were very specific. Not just in the types of work we did, but in how we positioned our bodies while performing each task. Everything, down to the way we stood, was important. I didn't know it then, but this was a method designed for the training of monks, and taught to my grandfather by his sifu, Zi Man and Chi Yat. It was hard work, and I complained all the time.

We had no running water on the farm, no plumbing, no irrigation system, and the nearest well was a quarter mile away, down the steep dirt path toward the village. To transport water, we used a six-wheeled, wooden cart with spoked, rubber tires. The buckets were made from large cookie tins, with lids removed and a one-by-one-inch stick fastened across the top to form a handle. The cart held twenty-four of these tin buckets. Making the water-trip down the hill was fun. My older brothers pushed the cart, and let the younger children jump on and ride. Such activity was forbidden by my father. It was all right to replace a piece of equipment because it wore out or broke down on the job. But it was unacceptable to break something while playing. Even so, when we had turned the bend and were out of sight of our house, we climbed on the cart. You could hear the giggling and the clacketty-clack of the buckets all the way down to the barge dock.

The first half of the water-fetching was my favorite, but the return trip could be most difficult. It took four of us—shoulders pressed against the cart's wooden panels, and legs churning through the dust and gravel—to push the twenty-four water-filled cookie tins up the hill.

There were two trips a day to the well—once in the morning and once in late afternoon. When pushing the cart home, we were instructed to use the "horse stance"—legs spread, knees slightly bent, hips flexed forward, elbows bent, palms flexed, and stomachs tight. And we employed the rhythmic dan tein breathing—in through the nose, out through the nose, expanding the diaphragm. This technique was a very important part of our t'ai chi training, but at the age of six I thought I had to breathe through my nose to keep flies out of my mouth.

The first water-trip was for the animals—one hundred pigs, about two thousand chickens, ducks, pigeons, and geese, six dogs, and a pond full of carp.

The pond, an artificial pool of fresh water ringed with watercress, needed aeration. So, three buckets-full were splashed into different spots marked by planks of wood. The younger children, with help from older siblings, stood on stools and emptied the tins from a height that made the biggest splashes.

We used ropes tied to the ends of long bamboo poles to carry water to the other animals. The heavy cookie tins were filled to the brim with water. We fastened the tin handles to hooks at the ends of each rope, then we'd place the bamboo poles across our shoulders, and lift. The carriers were made with different rope lengths—short for younger children, long for the older ones. Balance was very important. Father instructed us to hold our stomachs tight, our backs straight, palms facing the sky to steady the poles, shoulders square, and as always breathe through the nose. Each step was measured, heel first, then toe—strong and deliberate. We knew that no one would be angry if we spilled the water. We just had to make the trip down the hill to the well alone to get more. I was always very careful.

When the animals were well watered, we marched back to the house for breakfast, then went to school. From 8:00 am to 11:30 am we learned to read, write, and speak in both English and Chinese. A one-room building served as the educational center of our village. During the morning hours children ages 6 to 12 sat on the long benches, each child supplied with slates, papers, and pencils. Older children received instruction in the afternoon, and adults met for town meetings after sunset.

When the school bell clanged, we headed back up the hill to our afternoon chores.

We raised ducks, geese, and chickens. Half of the eggs we sold, the other half we kept to replenish the stock. Every day we had to clean dozens of pens and cages, and change the water.

Pigeons, a delicacy in many Hong Kong restaurants, sold for a very good price, and were a major part of our farm's income. We raised the chicks until they were fledglings, grouped them into A, B, or C grades, and took them to market.

The pigeons lived in a cage as big as small house, with room for each pigeon to have its own nest. I still remember the day my father taught me to clean the pigeon cage.

We carried water tins along the narrow footpath that led to the pigeon house. Father took me by the hand, and walked me through the screened door of the noisy building. Birds fluttered over us, making the interior look like a blur of feathers and wings.

"It stinks!" I yelled, trying to pull my hand away.

My father held tight. "It is supposed to smell," he said. "What we feed them comes out. What we feed you comes out, too." He laughed. "You smell worse."

I punched him, but his tight muscles made my fist hurt. "I won't go in there," I told him. "You go. I will wait here."

Father opened the door and dragged me in. "You are old enough now."

"I am only six!" I yelled. "I am not tall enough to reach the nests. That's why I can't help get the pigeons ready for market."

"Here," he said, handing me a small metal shovel. "See the stool in the corner? You use that to reach the top poles. All the white stuff has to be scraped off, then rinsed with water. Then you must sweep out the mess, and put it all in this bucket."

"No," I said. "I am too young."

Father pushed me into the cage, walked out, and latched the door. "I'll be back soon. Do it fast."

"It stinks in here," I cried.

"That will change," he said, walking back down the path. "After a while you won't smell anything. Just get it done." He kept walking, and didn't look back.

I sat on the white-speckled ground, pigeon waste splattered everywhere. I looked around, then at the locked door. The only way out was to work.

I learned many lessons while I cleaned that cage. As I slouched in the midst of fallen feathers and sticky droppings, something hit the top of my head. I looked up, mouth open. That was the first lesson. Even in here, where it stinks, breathe through your nose.

That cage was really dirty. I scraped for hours, tip-toeing on the stool to reach the highest wooden roosting dowels. When pigeon poop is dry, it sticks like glue. My arms and wrists ached.

I complained to my father that evening, and he said, "Cleaning the pigeons' cage is one of the most important jobs." I could hear the crackling of the fire over Father's soft voice. "That is how the monks trained in the olden days."

"They had pigeons?" I asked.

"Oh, yes," he said. "They learned to build their energy, their strength, by cleaning the cages. When you hold the shovel, it makes your wrist strong."

I rubbed my arms, and listened.

"It will help you when you learn the kung fu techniques. You'll see."

I tried not to complain, but I didn't care if cleaning up after those filthy birds was noble or important. I hated that chore. And kung fu now began to sound like work.

The other animals were not much easier to tend. We had to wash down the pigs, and clean their pens. That was difficult, but I got to work with my brothers and sisters, and that always made the jobs seem much less difficult.

One day, my little brother Luk Chun Ming and I were helping our older brother Luk Chun Yuen clean the pigs. When pigs see water, they squeal and run.

Chun Yuen, who was two years older than me, said, "Stand by the gate, and make sure that the pigs don't get out."

We stood sentry, proudly guarding the gate using the chi kung "horse stance," with hands out in front of us. "Be strong," he said. "Keep them in the fence."

We weren't going to let any of them out, not even the littlest one.

Chun Yuen grabbed a bucket, and tossed the water over the back of one of the largest pigs. He jumped, and bolted for the gate where my younger brother stood. Chun Ming crouched lower, planting his feet, and making himself solid. The pig picked up speed, lowered his head like a goat, and plowed into Chun Ming. Both of them screamed. I couldn't tell which sound came from the pig. Chun Ming flew through the air, legs and arms flailing in all directions, and landed upside-down in the food trough. The pig galloped toward the vegetable garden, and I fell over laughing. I got into much trouble for laughing and not helping my poor brother out of the slop. But it was the funniest thing I had ever seen.

Every late afternoon, Father came up the hill pushing a cart filled with discarded food. He had an agreement with the restaurant owners of the village to pick up their scraps for our pigs. Feeding the fish was easy, the ducks and chickens took very little time. But feeding the pigs was torture.

If you give pigs cold food, they become sick. So each day, no matter what time of year, we chopped vegetables and mixed them with the fat, rice, and restaurant scraps Father brought from the village. We heated the food in a wok, about 6 feet in diameter, over an open fire. Four of us at a time took turns stirring the mass of slop with large wooden paddles. We stood on a thin ledge that circled the wok. Father always told us, "Work is the best teacher." He said, "When you do a job correctly—use the right stance, the right technique—the work will teach your body to be strong, and your mind to focus." We had to focus or fall into the hot slop, and the scalding wok beneath it.

Everything we did seemed a part of our t'ai chi training, a new exercise. Each chore had great meaning, a secret reason for the difficulty and strain.

Gathering the firewood to heat the pigs' food was such a chore, a form of training. Below our farm, at the base of the long hill, there was a boatyard where they made wooden junks, the big ones used for fishing. At the center of the boatyard stood a huge two-story mill with a large circular saw for trimming logs to make the hull planks for the junks. The boss of the mill gave my father access to the mill, permission for his sons to gather wood chips for our wok fire.

This was a job for the older boys. When I was little, I heard stories about their experiences dodging the chips and wood chunks the saw spat at them. The stories were of heroism and courage, and on days I had to clean the pigeon cage, I practiced dodging the poop, and pretended it was flying wood. I begged to go with them to the mill, but they said I might get hurt.

Eventually I grew up, and it was my turn to fight the "dragon" saw for my treasure of wood chips.

I walked down the hill following my brothers, who pulled a small wagon. There was a drone in the distance. It grew louder as we walked. When we arrived at the gate, the guard looked down at me and said, "Who's this one? He's the runt, yes?" I was eleven years old. Everybody laughed. I started to get upset and then I saw it, the source of the noise we had heard growing as we approached—the two-story building, the cavernous square saw-housing, a giant pile of debris, and sawdust and wood chips hurling through the air like brown fireworks. I suddenly missed my little pigeon house.

The guard waved us through the gate, and we walked toward the mill. The saw was screaming, a roaring scream. I could hear the wood screaming. But if I screamed, it would be silent in comparison.

My brothers got right to work. They ran in and out of the swirling chaos, bobbing up and down and sideways. I stood in shock.

"Come here, Chun Chi!" my brothers yelled. "Help us!"

Thick logs moved slowly along conveyer belts to the second floor of the mill, where they met the whirring metal teeth. I tried to find the rhythm of each blast from the saw. There was none. It was constant explosion. We ducked and dodged as chunks of wood, some larger than my 11-year-old body, flew through the air. My oldest brother moved so quickly. I would reach for a piece of wood, and he'd grab it and toss it into the wagon. I ran around confused in the sawdust for a while, and I didn't contribute anything to the mound of wood gathered on the wagon. It was almost filled.

I ran back into the storm, determined to add to our wood harvest. A chunk, about two feet long, flew past my head, and fell near my right foot. I reached down, grabbed it, and ran toward the wagon. I stopped to throw my prize onto the pile, when I felt something hit my head. Everything went black, but I could feel my body move in slow motion, like falling through thick mud.

I remember the jostling of the wagon on the way home, and the faint, concerned tones of my brothers' voices.

When my father came to my sleeping mat to see how I felt, he said, "You are still young. You shouldn't have gone to the mill. That is a job for quick reflexes and alertness. You must move like lightning, and watch everything, on all sides." He lifted the damp cloth and examined the welt behind my ear. "You are lucky to have such a hard head, stubborn, inside and out." He rubbed my shoulder, and stood to leave. "You are a strong boy, a good worker. You don't have to do this job just yet. Let the older boys gather the wood, for a little while longer."

I loved my father. His every word made the best sense. He was so wise. I slept well that night, and I didn't have to work at all the next day. I changed my attitude after the flying wood experience. Being quick and agile became my goal. I would meet the saw dragon again, and this time I would be the victor.

So I began to practice moving like lightning, until three weeks before my twelfth birthday. After my accident at the mill I experienced short bouts of dizziness. I never told anyone, but sometimes I had to hold onto something to keep from falling.

Like the other farms in the village, we had an outside bath house with a narrow, steep-sided metal tub. Many people had accidents because of the slippery tub walls.

One evening as I stepped into the heated water, everything began to spin. I lost my footing, and crashed backward. My spine snapped, and a warm sensation draped my body. I lay face up, arched over the tub side. I must have let out a cry, because my brothers came in and carried me to the house.

Father took me to a hospital in Hong Kong where they took x-rays, and doctors poked and pulled on my back and neck. There must have been ten nurses and doctors in the room. They all told us that I would be fine in two weeks.

But two weeks passed, and still the doctors said I would be fine, only things did not get better. My feet and legs would go numb and turn purple, my head ached all the time, and the pain in my back made it impossible to stand or walk. Then the doctors revised their prognosis and said I would probably have to be in a wheelchair.

Finally, weak from the pain, and crying in frustration, I asked my father to teach me the healing chi kung.

"Oh," he said. "Finally, you ask."

"What do you mean?"

"I can only help you if you ask."

"It will heal me, yes, Father?"

"Oh, yes," he said. "You will feel the difference instantly."

Father asked me to roll over onto my stomach, close my eyes, and do my dan tein breathing. I never felt his hands touch my skin, but I sensed the warm, gentle prickling of his energy—his chi—penetrate my back, into my spine.

"Relax," he said. "Do not fight the sleep."

As he said that, I drifted into the most restful night's sleep I can remember.

Father prescribed a series of exercises I could do while lying in bed. He told me how many times to do each one, how long to work, and how long to rest. And every evening, when he arrived home from Hong Kong, he would ask me how I did. Each night I felt a little better, and each night he would prescribe a new set of exercises for the following day.

It took some time before my father finally said that my body was healed. Although I felt better while I did the exercises, he kept saying, "Feeling good is a sign that you are on the path to recovery, but it does not always mean that you have recovered completely. Health is a moving element of life. You are either spiraling upward into good health, or downward into bad health. When the body is well, the chi moves freely through the meridians, and can instantly heal any illness. You must keep the meridians open, so the chi can work its magic."

Father finally pronounced me healed a few days before Chinese New Year. In Chinese tradition, it didn't matter if the year just ending was good or bad. Everything had to be made fresh for the new year. It was time to change your world in preparation for the good luck of a new start. If you made a profit with your work, you rejoiced and brought the prosperity into your home in the form of new clothes, shoes, and furniture. It was like a harvest of good luck, a time of thanksgiving.

Father always bought us new shoes and new clothes. The house received a new coat of paint and some new furnishings. He instructed the carpenter to complete all repairs before the celebration began.

Early on the morning before he made his annual shopping trip into Hong Kong, my father came to my room. Even in my half-sleep, I could feel his presence. My brothers and I slept on mats lined up side-by-side along the east wall of the house. As I lay on my stomach, I felt a tingling sensation move from the base of my head, down my spine. "Roll over, " my father said, quietly. I did so.

"It's too early. I am sleeping."

"Shhh. Lie still," he said. He placed his hands about eight inches above the center of my chest. I felt a shiver as he slowly surveyed my meridian channels for blocks. Father always examined me in the early morning. As he said, "It is when your chi is quiet, like a sleeping house. The hallways and rooms are open, free of people and obstruction."

My father's chi had a distinctive feel, like a low-grade vibration that resonated through my body.

He moved his hands into the air above my torso, then down my legs, up to my shoulders and along my arms, never touching my body. He said, "Your channels are open. You are fine. Your strength will come back even stronger now. Resume your training." This meant that I could do my full range of responsibilities, like gathering water and wood chips, and cleaning the pigeon cages. I wasn't excited about that.

When I was 16 years old my mother fell ill. She simply said it was time for her to go. Father couldn't help her. We didn't understand why, but it was her decision. She had dreamed her next life, and wanted to go there. She called each of us to her bedside, and gave instructions. To my older sister she said, "You are the mother now. Be kind to my children. They are no longer your brothers and sisters. They are your children. Love them, protect them."

I was far from the bed and could not hear her words, but I know for certain she said this, because later when my sister got angry with me she would say, "I wish Mother were alive. There was a reason she was your mother, not me. Now I must honor my promise and put up with you."

My turn came, and Mother beckoned me to kneel beside her. She held her hand out on the bed. I remember the room being dark, and I could not tell if her eyes were open. Her breathing came shallow. I knelt, and when I put my hand in hers, I noticed that her soft, gentle palms had grown cold and rough. "You, my boy, are so much like your father. But you are too impatient," she said. "One day, you will become a t'ai chi master, and carry on when your father is gone." She let out a sigh. "It will take you a long time to tame the tiger in you, and calm your aggressive spirit. Promise me that you will carry on your father's work. Train hard, and study the t'ai chi."

In Chinese astrology, I was born in the year of the metal tiger, a very strong sign with a tendency to be a fearless and fiery fighter. My mother was always saying, "Calm down." "Be patient." "Relax." Her admonitions didn't make sense to me when I was young. The time I hurt my back, she said, "See, you must slow down. You do not listen to your mother, so your body will force you to be calm."

My mother refused to go to the hospital. She wanted to die in her bed. She was a forceful woman, strong-willed and insistent. But we were glad it would happen at home. We could not bear to have her away from us.

On a cold, windy night when gusts climbed the hill to our house and slammed against the wooden walls, my mother closed her eyes for the last time. She tried to open them once, raising her brows to lift the weight of her heavy lids, but she didn't succeed. Father stroked her white hair. The children knelt around the edges of the bed. Then Mother's soul left us. I think she got up out of her old body, and went outside and joined the wind.

My younger sister reached out and touched Mother's foot, then she shrunk away, sobbing, and ran into the other room. We all wept, for a long time. The room turned humid with tears.

Aside from the cries of her children and the blustering wind outside, Mother's life escaped her body like the a butterfly lifting from its cocoon.

The impact of her subtle strength and the ache her absence left in our family made my promise to her my life's goal. From the moment of her death, I dedicated myself to training in the complete art of t'ai chi.

Father was my sifu. After we finished the farm work, my brothers and I would walk down the hill to Father's school for lessons in t'ai chi ch'uan, kung fu, chi kung, and feng shui. Because of my youth and speed, I excelled (and had the greatest interest) in the most physical aspect of t'ai chi—the martial art of kung fu. I trained constantly, incorporating the breathing, postures, movement patterns, and concepts of weight transference into every aspect of my life. I found that my work at home went smoother, almost effortless. Gathering wood chips became an exercise in peripheral awareness and agility—ducking, dodging, and parrying.

I studied hard under my father's tutelage, and by the summer of my eighteenth year, I advanced to the position of single master. Within the carefully guarded secrets of the master's ceremony is a pledge given by the advancing student to Cheung San Fung, the founder of t'ai chi. I had to promise never to use my skills to damage or harm, never to fight or act in aggression.

After the ceremony, Father took me to the path that led to Devil's Hill. "You know," he said. "When I was training, my father told me that the sifu determines when a student is ready for advancement. You understand the skills of kung fu, but now it is time to train in the other disciplines. Tomorrow you begin work in chi kung."

I couldn't believe what he was saying. "Father," I said. "I am a master now. I want to go to Hong Kong and compete. I want to learn kick boxing."

By the time we'd reached the summit of Devil's Hill, our conversation was an argument. Father refused to allow me to go into the city's martial arts district. "Those people are ruthless," he said. "You are not ready."

"I am a master!" I yelled. "You are my sifu. You declared that I had mastered the kung fu. Isn't your training enough for me to beat opponents in competition?"

"Yes," he said. "You will win, if that is what you choose to do. But remember your pledge to Cheung San Fung. No fighting. Only use your kung fu for defense."

"There is no good having this skill and not test how good I am," I said. "Are you afraid the training from you might not be enough? I'm young and strong. I can beat anybody."

"It is true you are young," Father said. "You have so much more to learn. You need to understand all the elements of t'ai chi."

"That's an excuse," I complained. "I'm ready and you know it!"

I remember that day, standing above the village, the day my father made me question the training I'd received all my life.

"Maybe you don't think I'm good enough to fight the people in Hong Kong!" I yelled. I'd lost my temper, as usual.

And Father remained calm. He turned toward the south, with his back to me, and took a deep breath. "You may go," he said, and he started down the hill.

I called after him, but he wouldn't look back. "Why did you bring me all the way up here?" I asked. He kept walking, one carefully placed step after the other.

The next day, my brothers Chun Yuen and Chun Ming boarded the Hong Kong ferry with me for our trip to the martial arts district. Father refused to accompany us. He stayed on the dock, and waited for the next boat to take him to work. He said nothing, no good luck or good fortune wishes. He kept his hands to his sides.

"I don't understand that old man," I said, watching his image get smaller as the boat pulled off into the channel.

My brothers said nothing. They were very excited, and were already at the other end of the boat looking toward the distant skyline of the city.

We must have walked for a mile through the crowded streets to get to the most famous kick boxing school in Hong Kong. We found the address in a long row of wooden warehouses. A small sign above a heavy door marked the do jo. It was an old school, and dimly lit. The air inside smothered us with the odor of years of triumph and glory. There were dozens of kick boxers, damp with sweat, leaping and striking at their opponents, chuffing forceful exhalations as they slammed to the mats.

A man in the middle of the large, open room yelled at us, "You, what you want?" He was older than the others, but very vibrant, a seasoned fighter.

My younger brother Chun Ming yelled back, "We are here to learn to kick box! This man is a kung fu master." He pointed at me.

The old man walked up, and all of the activity on the mats stopped. "Who?" he questioned. "You?" He laughed at me. "OK, get in the ring. Let's see what kind of master you are."

I pulled off my shirt.

"How are you going to fight?" Chun Yuen asked. "You don't know how to kick box. That's why we came here."

"I'll just do what I am trained for," I said. "All I know is Father's kung fu."

"Do you think it's enough?" Chun Ming asked.

"If it's not, I will learn something about kick boxing, " I said, and I walked onto center mats below a cluster of dangling naked light bulbs.

I bowed to the old man. He bowed back. "I am the sifu here," he said. "Only I determine who is a master." He undid his shirt and began to strip it off.

We circled, facing each other—a sinewy, smooth-skinned 18 year old and a weathered fighter baring a collection of scars, the rough trophies of a history of brutal matches.

I remembered Father's counsel, "You are impatient. Calm yourself. Let all opponents make the first move. To defend from a solid base is the best position."

I broadened my stance and lowered my center of gravity. "Wait, wait," I thought.

The old man quickly stepped forward, swinging his leg in a wide arch toward my head. I moved with more instinct than planning, placing my right foot forward and pivoting away from the oncoming blow. I swept my arms in one, single upward swoop, and deflected the kick, while allowing my opponent's momentum and force to twist him awkwardly around. Then, for the split-second his side was exposed, I hit him square in the ribs just above his black belt, and knocked him to the ground.

As he lay on the mat, gasping for breath, I knelt to help him. "Get out!" he hissed, waving me away. "Get out of here!"

The other students, hearing their sifu's command, moved toward me. I couldn't see my brothers in the crowd of sweating boxers. Then I saw the door to the school open. Light from the outside broke the dismal gloom of the artificially lit do jo. I pushed through the group, sprinted to the door, and ran with my brothers through the rows of warehouses. We didn't stop until we were back at the dock.

On the way home, Chun Yuen asked, "What moves did you use? It looked like the horse stance and then everything happened so fast, and I couldn't see through the crowd."

I parried his kick with the "Wild Horse Parting Mane" move, then hit him with the "Fist Under the Elbow."

"It was great!" said Chun Ming. He swung his arms in the air, mimicking kung fu movements and shadow boxing. He was 14 years old, and easily excited.

Chun Yuen and I sat on the dock—our feet dangling over the edge—while Chun Ming danced

"I guess we can't go back there to learn kick boxing," Chun Yuen said.

"No," I said. "I don't think I'm interested anymore."

"Why?" he asked. "Don't you want to be in the martial arts?"

"I beat the master of one of Hong Kong's most prestigious kick boxing schools with two of Father's kung fu moves. The martial arts have nothing to teach me. I think I'll study to be a double master."

"In Father's school?" he asked.

"Yes," I said. I was hoping that Father would take me back into the school after my rudeness on Devil's Hill.

"So you become a double master," Chun Ming chimed. "What good is that? You won't know how to compete. There are no jobs in Hong Kong that advertise 'Needed: double kung fu master.' It's a waste of time. What do you have to gain?"

"The staff," I said.

Both brothers stared at me. Chun Ming sat down on the worn wood-plank dock. "Grandfather's staff?" he said. "You don't mean Grandfather's staff. Father will never give it to you. Of all his possessions, that is his favorite. He says it's magic, full of chi. He says it's hundreds of years old, used by generations of siu lum monks."

"I know," I said. "That is why I want it."

"You won't get it," Chun Yuen said. "He'll hand it down to the oldest, not you. Who are you to get something like that?"

The ferry horn sounded as it eased into the slip. We stood up and headed for the gate.

"I am a master now, and will be a double master soon. Then Father will see that I am worthy of the staff. He will give it to me. I will earn it."

After my Hong Kong kick boxing experience, life moved in a sequence of lessons. There was only one constant interference with my training regimen—Father. His instruction on the feng shui, the complex study of magnetic fields and chi movement, left me confused. And his explanations of the esoteric healing techniques of chi kung struck no chords of recognition for me. I was 18 years old, and during that turbulent time I felt physically superior to my aging father. The concepts of healing and restoring youthful vigor meant little. I was strong and healthy, an impatient learner. I grew bored with the slow, concentrated movements of t'ai chi ch'uan and chi kung, and the tedious theories of feng shui. I still wanted to fight!

On some days the tensions flared. I lost my temper in violent displays, and lashed out at my father. As I look back to those years, I understand my reactions, for I was an independent, headstrong young man. Father said, "You are so loud in your impatience that you can't hear the subtle wisdom in the wind, or the water." These were references to feng shui, which means "wind water." He was talking about the energies that surround us, those we generate, and those that are generated in the earth and sky. Thinking of such invisible things was very difficult. I struggled with the concentration needed for the exercises, sloshing through their slow movements like a champion swimmer forced to wade across a pond instead of swim it. To stop my active kung fu practice and have to meditate or observe some bird my father pointed to as an illustration of balance only made me angry.

Two years went by. I kept going through my father's lessons even though I detested them. And I had not reached the level of double master. One day, I exploded.

My two closest brothers had gone into Hong Kong to pursue careers. One was a bouncer in the black market and the other a junior body builder. Father nagged at them to continue their study of the healing arts. One evening as the three us—Chun Yuen, Chun Ming, and myself—sat on a knoll on the edge of our garden and complained about Father's persistence, we realized that we had never seen him actually fight. "Maybe it's all just rumor," Chun Ming said. "Maybe the old men in this village are making the stories up. Have you seen him fight?"

Chun Yuen and I looked at each other, then at Chun Ming. "No," I said.

"Then how do we know all this stuff he's teaching us is true?" Chun Ming asked.

I thought. "I know that the kung fu I learned is good," I said. "I know I can fight."

"Yes, but all of that healing stuff," Chun Yuen said. "Did he save Mother?"

I jumped to Father's defense. "No," I said. "But he healed my back when the doctors in Hong Kong said nothing could be done. They said I was going to be in a wheelchair."

"But did he heal you, or did you heal yourself?" Chun Ming asked.

"This is stupid," I said. "I hate the training, but I think Father knows what he is talking about."

"Do you want to spend the next ten years studying this?" Chun Yuen asked. "You should come to Hong Kong with us. The city is exciting, and there are women, many women." He made a naughty gesture and we all laughed.

The deep purple light of evening was slowly giving way to night when we heard Father call from the house. "There he is again," Chun Ming said. "Do you think we'll have to put up with the lectures about Grandfather and t'ai chi again?"

"I'm sick of it!" I said. "I'm sick of all of it."

"Then come with us tomorrow," Chun Yuen urged. "Come into the city. I can get you a job."

"I don't want to work in the black market," I said. "And I don't want to spend my days in a gym to make my body big."

"Just come with us," they said. Both my brothers put their arms around my shoulders. "We will tell Father your training is over, and you have decided to go with us."

"When?" I asked. "When will we tell him?"

"Tomorrow morning," Chun Yuen said. "We'll tell him after breakfast."

We rose early, before the roosters, and did the chores quickly. Breakfast was quiet. Father, looking tired, sat at the head of the low table. Chun Yuen spoke first. "Father," he said. "Chun Ming and I are taking Chun Chi to Hong Kong with us today. We are going to get him a job in the city."

Father looked up from his bowl of rice. "No," he said quietly. "Chun Chi will stay here and study."

Chun Ming started to speak. "We've . . ."

Father looked up again. "No more!" he said. "There is nothing more to say." He stood and walked to the door. "Chun Ming and Chun Yuen, go to Hong Kong. Chun Chi, you come with me."

That is what finally made something in my core ignite. "No!" I yelled. "I am done with studying. I am going with them today."

Father turned and walked outside.

Our attack was sudden and unplanned. It was more a rage than a fight. We attacked Father from behind, his three young, very strong sons. I lunged first, aiming a two-fisted blow to the middle of his back. The rest happened so quickly that some of the details are lost, even in the slow motion of memory. Father stepped wide, stretching his left leg to the side. As my momentum carried me forward, I tripped on his foot. He grabbed my head, twisted his torso, and planted his elbow between my nose and mouth. I felt a numbing blast radiate from the blow as I fell. I don't remember hitting the ground, but I tasted the salty warmth of blood in my mouth. I looked up. Chun Yuen and Chun Ming attacked Father at the same time. He fought back like a strong wind, twisting and contorting to deliver solid hits to each of his sons. The fight was short. In a matter of seconds my brothers lay beside me. Blood covered all of our faces.

Father said, "Chun Chi. I will see you at the school. Clean yourself off. Chun Yuen and Chun Ming, go to work." Father walked down the dirt path, his feeble gait disguising the strength and power he carried with him.

"Are you all right?" I asked my brothers.

"Yes," they said, but they remained prostrate on the ground. Chun Ming started to laugh. "You ask us if we are okay, and you are the one missing a tooth."

I felt my mouth. "No!" I said. There was a gap where my left incisor used to be.

"I think the old man has given you a trophy," said Chun Yuen.

"I guess so."

I respected Father deeply after that. And I never complained or argued, for whenever there were moments of doubt, I always had my missing tooth to remind me of the skill Father had attained in the mastery of chi—the skill that I hoped would someday be mine as well.

At the age of 21, I finally left the farm and my father's school. I was going to Hong Kong to begin my adult life. I had completed all of the lessons, and on the day I left home Father said, "Someday what you've learned will become a part of who you are, and you will return to become a double master."

The years in the city left me empty. I joined the Hong Kong police, but the darkness associated with the job depleted my energy. I left the force after only six months, and signed on to become a merchant marine. My travels took me around the Orient and South Pacific. On board ship, I taught the sailors kung fu. We held classes on the open deck, fighting each other while battling the pitch and roll of the ship. I honed my skills in all four aspects of t'ai chi during the long voyages from port to port. I taught whoever would sit long enough to listen. Even the captain of one of our vessels let me adjust his cabin according to the principles of feng shui. I practiced t'ai chi ch'uan on the bow of the ship as the sun set on the South China Sea, and under a chandelier of stars in a moonless sky while enroute to Australia. I taught chi kung and t'ai chi ch'uan classes in London, Seattle, New York, Rio, Melbourne, and Acapulco.

I grew up during these years as a merchant marine. I had traveled around the world, and seen the beauty and drama each land afforded. And one clear morning while docked in Auckland, New Zealand, I knew it was time to return to my father, and finish my training.

I terminated my contract, and purchased an airplane ticket to Hong Kong. With duffel bag slung over my shoulder, and passport in hand, I boarded the China Air flight for my first experience on an airplane. I had no idea what to expect. I had never been so excited.

The doors were sealed, the engines wound into a high-pitched roar, and we began to move down the runway. My seat was near the back of the plane. The noise shook the whole cabin, and the vibration churned my body as the plane lifted from the tarmac into a slow climb to the clouds.

I thought of my promise to my mother, to carry on Father's teaching. And I thought about my name, Luk Chun Chi, which means "a person who goes to a foreign country to share knowledge." Finally my name correlated with my promise, my mission. It all made sense to me. I would go home, complete my training, and venture out into the world to pass on the teachings of Grandfather's monks.

The plane ascended, then leveled. Flight attendants made their first beverage pass, offering soft drinks, water, and tea. My body buzzed with the hum of the engines, and soon I was asleep. There were no dreams, just the numbing blackness of complete rest.

I must have slept for hours. Dinner had been served, and the passengers were now enthralled in a Chinese martial arts movie that flashed above the plane's darkened tunnel of seats before me. I stood up, and walked to the stewardess station. "Do you have some tea?" I asked.

"Oh, yes," a young Chinese woman replied. "Where are you sitting? I will bring it to you."

I returned to my seat, and in moments I was sipping tea, and drifting in and out of another nap.

We were about an hour away from Hong Kong when the plane jolted and bounced, then jolted again.

"The captain has turned on the fasten seat belt sign," a female voice warned. "Please make sure your seat belts are securely fastened."

The plane lurched again, then bounced. It was like riding the water wagon down our hill at home. The passengers around me held tight to their seat arms, and near the front of the plane a baby started crying. Again a female voice chimed on the P. A. system, "The captain says that we'll be out of this turbulence very soon. Please remain calm and in your seat."

A woman, sitting a few rows in front of me, started screaming. "Help! Somebody help me!"

Over the scalloped rows of seats I could see her, standing over another passenger seated next to her. She called to the flight attendants, "It's my husband. He's having a heart attack. Help me!"

The plane continued with its bumping gyrations as several flight attendants quickly made their way to the hysterical woman's seat. Other passengers leaned and gawked, a bobbing field of heads craned to watch the drama.

I didn't know exactly what I could do, but I felt myself loosen the clamp on my seat belt, and rise. I walked down the aisle, swerving with the motion of the plane, and asked one of the attendants if I could help.

"Are you a doctor?" she asked.

"No," I said. "I am a chi kung master. I know I can help this man."

They cleared a path for me. I leaned in. Slumped over in his chair was an elderly man in his late 60s. His wife sobbed.

I took her hand, and looked into her eyes. "I can help him," I said. She fell back into her seat. Two flight attendants eased her away from us, and down the aisle to the back of the plane.

The man was still conscious, but his lips were purple. He was losing strength. I had helped heal sailors' sprained ankles and sore muscles, but I didn't know if I had the skill or power to help this man.

I closed my eyes, brought chi energy into my body, up through my meridians, and into my hands. Placing one hand on his forehead and another on his chest, I pushed my chi into his body. "Breathe with me," I told him. I pushed chi down into the meridians that served his heart, and then radiated it throughout his system. I could feel many blocks.

"Look at my forehead," I told the man. "Keep focused on me."

The man relaxed, but I could feel him concentrating. "Keep breathing with me," I told him. "Your breath and mine will join. Watch me and breathe when I do, like I do." I made sure that my rhythm was slow and consistent. Although he was weak, he kept time with me, inhaling and exhaling. I sensed him getting a little stronger. I focused on the heart meridians, massaging the blocks with concentrated chi. An illness like his would take years to heal and correct. For now, I just wanted to keep him alive until we landed in Hong Kong.

I worked on the man for a long while, keeping him breathing and in a state of high concentration. One of the flight attendants came to me and asked, "Is there anything I can do?"

"Get him some water. No ice. It needs to be room temperature."

The captain's voice came on the loud speaker, "We are making our final approach into Hong Kong International. Please remain in your seats."

"What is your name?" I asked the man.

"Robert," he said in a weak voice. "Robert O'Donnell from Auckland."

I smiled, and he closed his eyes and smiled back.

"Keep your eyes open," I said. "Let's stay focused until the doctor comes to get you, okay?"

He lifted his lids, and nodded.

An airport doctor boarded the plane as soon as the doors were open, and they took old Robert to the hospital.

I had not told anyone I was coming home. No one met me at the airport. I took a taxi to the dock, caught the ferry to our village, then started to climb the hill to our farm.

Everything was different. The lower portion of the hill had been graded, and new cement homes were under construction. The farm was overgrown, and our house, which I could see from the bottom of the dirt path, leaned in disrepair.

I ran the remaining distance. Our garden was gone, replaced by the beginnings of a wooden frame house. Nestled against the hillside, where the pigeon house used to be, stood a tall electric tower.

I went to the front door of our old house, and pushed it open. The entry-room lay bare except for the debris of neglect strewn across the floor: yellowed Chinese newspapers, broken dishes, a wicker chair without a seat. The place echoed with emptiness.

The sun was setting, so I turned toward the village. Tall, new buildings dotted the landscape. The other farms in the lower valley had disappeared, their fields divided into house lots. I spotted the roof of my father's t'ai chi school in the distance, and headed down the hill toward it.

Light from an electric bulb glowed from the open double doors of the school, and I caught the familiar smell of incense as I climbed the stairs. Father stood in the middle of the floor, surrounded by a large group of elderly people bending and turning through the t'ai chi ch'uan movements. He looked up and saw me in the doorway.

We all generate our own chi energy, and mine warmed my body with a powerful resonance of joy when I saw Father smile. There was such love emanating from that weathered old face. He walked into my arms, and I felt his strength, his heart, his intense power.

"You went to the farm?" he asked.

"Yes," I said. "What happened?"

"I sold it," he said with a smile. "Lots of money, and now, not so much work."

We both laughed. "I was actually looking forward to doing the chores," I said.

"There are always chores," he said. "This building needs a new roof, new lights, new steps, a new walkway, a new hall . . ."

I hugged him again.

We spent the rest of the evening in his new home, a small, two-bedroom house adjacent to the school. I heard about all of my brothers and sisters and their families, their jobs, their woes and their happiness. I told him about my travels, all of my teaching experiences, and the man on the plane.

He was most interested in the man on the plane. "And you elevated his chi with your own?" he asked.

"Yes."

"Afterward, did you feel stronger? Were you proud? Did it make you feel good to help him?"

"It feels good to help. But I was not proud. I am happy to do what I can for other people. Afterward I felt weaker. When the doctor came and they took the man from the plane, I stood by myself for a while and did the dan tien breathing to restore my chi."

Father nodded. He seemed deep in thought.

As we prepared to retire, he asked me, "Are you home to complete your training?"

"Yes," I said. "I have come to earn Grandfather's staff."

He laughed. "You think you have the right to such an honor?"

"I think I can earn that right. The honor will be your decision to bestow, as you think best."

I stayed with Father through the year, repairing the school building. Every nail hammered was a lesson in the flow of chi, every board placed a study in feng shui. My formal training took on a new beauty, an ecstasy in learning, and understanding through physical practice.

One day my father came to the back of the school building where I was nailing loose boards into a wall. "I have something for you," he said. He motioned for me to follow. He carried a large bag over his right shoulder. In his left hand he held Grandfather's staff. He said he used it only when he felt weak.

We walked for a long time, through the narrow streets of the modern village, past home sites that were now office buildings, farms that became tracts of houses. "Are we going to Devil's Hill?" I asked.

"Yes and no," Father said. We walked to the path we'd climbed years before. Father started up Devil's Hill first.

I followed closely behind. "Do you need help with the bag?" I asked. He didn't answer.

When we reached the top of the hill, Father found a place to sit with a clear view of the harbor and village below. He sat cross-legged, and placed the staff in front of him. The bag he lay on the ground to his right.

"Sit," he said, pointing to a spot on the other side of the staff. "Face me."

I did. I considered the feng shui of this spot. Father calculated everything before he asked anyone to do anything. I had experience to know that this old man, this person who had healed me and taught me to heal others, had a purpose for everything. His instructions always took into account direction, position, posture, activity, psychology.

"The village is changing very quickly," he said. "There is no hope of stopping it, and I have no reason to try. It is all for the best, all for the learning of those who participate in the growth. I am 78 years old, and it is much more enjoyable to watch others struggle with their lessons than get involved with them."

He fumbled with the bag, and pulled out some scrolls, incense, and matches. "You are ready to advance to double master," he said. He lit the incense sticks and set them upright in the ground. He didn't look at me. "You have proven yourself through your travels and classes, through your healing successes and your willingness to learn. There is nothing else you can learn from me. Your choices in life will teach you the rest."

He leaned forward and picked up the staff. He said, "There is one test you need to perform. I have told you the story about Grandfather lifting the staff with his two fingers." He inhaled deeply as he stood.

He was holding the staff between his thumb and forefinger. He waved the staff through the air with ease. I watched this miracle as though I were looking back through time, to an illustration of the family legend of my grandfather. "This is what I want you to do," Father said. He handed me the staff and sat back down. "It is all done with chi."

"I haven't practiced with this," I said. "I can't lift it now."

"Probably not," he said. "I know when my students are ready. And I do not think you will pass this test."

"Then why ask it of me?"

"Because you have always known that I would ask you some-day—if you persisted in your lessons—to lift the staff with your fingers. The challenge was always meant to come. Now you have it. Lift the staff."

I unfolded my legs and stood. The staff is 8 feet long, of very dense teak. I held it in both hands, like a long baseball bat.

"Close your eyes," Father said. "You know the story about the monk Zi Man. You know his instructions to Grandfather."

I closed my eyes, imagining Zi Man sitting before me. I inhaled and brought the chi in through my arms, into my hands, and joined with the staff. It became part of my body, an elongated arm, and extended lever. I held it with one hand and positioned my other thumb and forefinger where Father had placed his. Then I let go my grip and tried with all my art and concentration to keep the heavy wood in the air with just my thumb and forefinger. I felt gravity gain momentum in the staff, like an iron ball inside it rolling downhill. It plunged to the ground.

My father nodded. Then he made a small smile that only lifted the corners of his mouth. "Try to hold it upright in one hand," he said.

I was able to do that. I focused and breathed again, and held the staff in my right hand only, at one end. I positioned the staff before me, straight and long into the air.

"Fine. That is an accomplishment," Father said. "Very few men could hold a staff like that. But it is a result more of physical strength than of chi. Try it again with only your fingers."

I repeated the movement. Again the staff pulled to the ground. It clunked against the hard earth and I felt a corresponding thump in my dan tien. "I am not ready," I said.

Father held up one of the scrolls and read silently for a moment. "You have earned the right to practice with the staff," he said. "You are a double master."

"I am?"

"Yes. The staff is yours. When you earn the right to practice with it, that means you have earned the staff. You have become a double master. Now you begin the training for triple master."

"So we will practice with the staff?"

"You will practice," said Father. "I have other students to teach." He put the scrolls and matches back in the bag and stood up. The incense he left burning in the ground. The smoke curled slowly in the windless air.

"And me?" I asked. "How will I learn to raise the staff?"

"What can I teach a double master?" my father said. "The world, the whole universe, is your sifu now."

What happened that day was the beginning of a new life for me. The staff had been handed down through three generations. Father had used it to fight off 60 men to protect his family and the village. But for me the staff would become something different—a symbol of my dedication not to fight, but to heal.

I had met in Hong Kong a beautiful woman named Mary, who was also a student of t'ai chi ch'uan. Soon we married. We wanted to leave Hong Kong and settle in the place the Chinese emigrants used to call the Gold Mountain: America.

When I told my father our plans he said I should take an English name, for the English-speaking students I would be teaching in America. He suggested Bond. Bond is also a Chinese word that means "foreign land." Father said, "Since you are going to a foreign land, and will be a foreigner to the people you meet there, it is a good name." We looked up the word in an English dictionary, and we found many definitions. The one I liked best was "something that causes parts or particles to adhere together or unite." That is very much a definition of what a master and teacher of chi does.

So Luk Chun Bond became my new name. Mary and I left Hong Kong in 1978. We traveled to many places, and then we came to Honolulu, where we live today. It was a spiritual journey for me because it has brought me to the best place to start my teaching. Where we live, in the city between the dark green mountains and the sky-blue ocean, is a powerful location. Two mornings a week we walk to a park near the famous volcano crater of Diamond Head, and there I conduct free classes in chi kung.

Through teaching I have learned. I find myself learning from all of life. My father was very correct (as usual) when he said that the universe would be my sifu.

Every day I see the workings of chi. I am gratified as I watch my students progress in their knowledge if its secrets. I watch them move through the exercises with increasing grace and strength. They are restoring their health. They seem to be growing younger, no matter how old they are. They tell me they feel better than they have felt in many years.

The magic of chi really works. Anyone who has worked with chi knows that by doing very simple exercises and eating foods that balance the yin and yang energies, your body will become stronger, your mind wiser, and you will feel more at ease with yourself and the world around you.

My students come from all over, not just Honolulu. People visiting the Islands often attend my classes, and many of them return, like seasonal birds to our little flock under the banyan trees. Later, I will tell you some of the wonderful stories of these students.

It is for my students that I have written this book. So many times they asked for a text to follow if they cannot come to class. But also I write for my mother, whom I promised that I would pursue a mission to carry on Father's teachings. And, of course, I write this for my father as well, the man who healed me and taught me to heal.

Confucius said, "The more we learn, the more we comprehend how little we know."

I have discovered that whenever I work with chi I learn its lessons all over again. This is something you will notice with this book. Each time you start an exercise or contemplate upon the meanings and presence of chi, it is a new beginning, a fresh start, no matter how advanced you have become in your lessons. Each time, your body will be invigorated. Your mind will expand. You will be able to move with more grace, lift things with more strength. New ideas will occur to you, tasks will be completed with greater ease, your focus will sharpen. Because of your growth in understanding and channeling chi, your fortunes will increase, you will notice beauty where you never thought to look before, love will bloom like a garden around you, and wonderful people will enter your life, attracted by your radiance. These things, too, I am learning and relearning, for I will always be a student progressing through the lessons that the universe brings me.

And though I have not yet been able to raise my grandfather's staff with only my thumb and forefinger, someday I will.

The Secret of the Enchanting Chi

I remember the first time I looked up the word *chi* in an English dictionary. I found chi, but it was pronounced KHY, and defined as "the 22nd letter in the Greek alphabet, written X."

This was very interesting for me. The Greek "khi" makes the shape for the basic chi posture, where a student stands with feet shoulder-width apart and back straight. In this position your legs and trunk form an X, or double triangle. Carpenters use the X in building because it is a very strong and balanced support structure.

Many centuries ago, Chinese philosophers and healers began to study the strange phenomena they had witnessed in nature. They marveled at how cranes and turtles could live so long, how plants were able to collect and move light, and how the human hand imparted the sacred touch of life. These men of ancient science understood that what governed such miracles was an invisible energy field called "chi."

Literally translated from Chinese to English, chi means "breath." But this breath is more than just air. It is air clarified by a particular spiritual light; it is the charged essence of life. In poetry, chi is the wind and stars, and it flows like a luminous stream through everything physical and metaphysical.

One time in his early training, my grandfather asked his sifu what chi looked like. It was just before bedtime, on a cloudless and moonless night. The two of them stood alone in the monastery courtyard.

"You see that river of stars?" the old man said. He pointed above the walls to the Milky Way. It spanned the whole sky, like a spangled arch. "Chi looks like that."

But then the next morning the sifu said, "Remember what I told you last night? Now I must tell you that chi is more than a stream of stars in the black sky. Chi also looks like that," he said. He pointed to the rising sun. "Chi is a ball of light that grows and shrinks and grows again, depending on how you see it in your imagination."

In fact, chi is all these things. Like the Greek chi, it is a support structure. It is the life force. It is light and every color in the spectrum. It is the recurring phenomenon of change that rules the dynamics of our world, an electromagnetic presence found in everything alive, including water and stone.

In Western cultures the concept of chi energy has been known by many names, and it has been studied for centuries. Astrology, meditation, positive thinking, massage therapy, holistic healing, and the observation of energy waves surrounding a person's body—the force field called the "aura"—all of these disciplines are rooted in chi.

The primary sources of chi are the universal energy showered on us from above, and the earth's nurturing elements rising from below. In ancient cultures all over the world, this duality is recognized in the mythical figures of father sky and mother earth.

Sky and earth form parallel curves. Their two forces converge, and where they meet, we live.

Chi encircles and penetrates our bodies. It is a charged mass that flows from the outside world to us, and which we project back into the environment. When we take the sky and earth chi into ourselves through vertical (dan tien or deep diaphragm) breathing, it courses along a series of power pathways called meridians.

The chi life force travels through the meridians, then branches into smaller and smaller channels to feed every cell in our bodies. As chi energy nourishes each cell, it elevates the cell's health and function.

In China, we divide chi into two distinct and opposing forces called yin and yang—dai yin, the passive, nutrient-rich earth; and tin yang, the potent, moving energy of heaven. Each has a tangible effect on us and our environment, and each is necessary for growth. But if not kept in balance, a dominance of either yin or yang has the potential to destroy.

Yin and yang are elements in harmonious opposition. They are depicted as a circle, divided in half by a wavy (sigmoid) line. One half is white, symbolizing the energy yang, and the other half is dark, symbolizing yin. A dot appears in the center of the bulbous section of each half—the white half (yang) with a dark "yin spot" and the dark half (yin) with a white "yang spot." This symbol serves as a reminder that these polar energies exist as blended and balanced, each surrounding and incorporating the other.

Think of yin and yang as two fish, circling one another in a mating ritual that produces life.

Yin and yang swirl constantly. The dynamic chi cycle affects, permeates, and nurtures all things—people, animals, plants, mountains, rivers, oceans, air, and space.

Chi is an essential substance often overlooked by Western doctors. Good health is achieved by maintaining and balancing the two basic life forces: yin, the meditative or quiet portion of our lives; and yang, the active portion. Any medical treatment will be enhanced and accelerated by chi therapy.

Balanced chi ignites a glow that radiates from the dan tien through the body to promote optimum health in much the same way nutrients and blood flow from the heart. We bring chi in by breathing.

Our bodies also create chi. The Chinese call this biological energy "jung chi," human-created chi. Thoughts, emotions, physical activities, and diet contribute to jung chi, which shines within us like an electric light.

When we are healthy our bodies balance yin and yang. The electrical current is strong. Organs and muscles work together to create an equilibrium, and then our light shines so brightly that its secret illumination extends into the air around us. Other people can sense it.

From the time we are born our bodies naturally produce jung chi. Babies instinctively breathe vertically. Watch any baby and you will see. Babies' tummies inflate when they breathe.

As we grow to adulthood, the very power of our growth, of cells renewing themselves and building the body outward, helps protect us. But while we age we encounter more and more problems. We become increasingly familiar with the external world. Our breathing patterns change, and we inhale too often with our lungs, expanding the chest instead of the abdomen. Our perceptions, beliefs, opinions, thoughts, stresses, and judgments can form blocks in the chi meridians and cause illness.

At times, our physical movements may bring an injury—a bruise, a scrape, a turned ligament—that results in meridian blocks.

Sometimes our diets, with over-processed foods and deficient vitamins, impede the vital life force.

A break in the chi flow—from outside or from our own jung chi—causes meridian blocks. Any meridian block will make our bodies unbalance, with the yin/yang energies unable to stimulate the internal organs. Our vibrancy lowers, hormone production becomes erratic, and illness finally ensues.

But we can clear the meridians at any time, and allow chi to surge uninterrupted. The body is designed to heal itself anyway. Once we open the meridians through concentration and even very little movement, the enlivened chi begins to charge each cell with energy and health.

I have worked with people of all ages, from children suffering attention deficit syndrome (too much yang energy), to sedentary adults experiencing the effects of heart disease, osteoarthritis, and diabetes (too much yin energy). As my students learn to control and move the chi into their meridians and channels, they report a delightful, tingling sensation and a feeling of overall well-being.

In this book, I will teach you the easiest and most effective chi kung exercises. These are the primary secrets of the ancient Chinese healing arts, the secrets of the enchanting chi. Learning and practicing these simple movements will bring peace, balance, and replenishing health to your life.

Feng Shui and the Human Body

The discipline of feng shui, an integral part of t'ai chi practice, is the study of chi pathways through a physical landscape—around mountains, down valleys, flowing with the course of rivers, riding the wind through the sky, and into every room of a building or house. The natural laws governing feng shui also apply to the dynamics of the human body, both in terms of chi pathways inside us and our position in relation to objects in our environment.

By bringing together the postures of chi kung exercises and the beneficial arrangements of feng shui, we can magnify the benefits. The precise location of our workout—the direction we face and our proximity to certain objects—is as important as performing the exercises correctly.

Translated from Chinese, feng shui means, "wind water." Both of these fluid elements are used as symbols for the movement patterns of chi. In nature, wind and water carry energy, like the rush of wind before a rain storm, or the gusts we feel when standing beside the crashing cascade of a waterfall. Like wind and water, chi moves in straight, powerful lines, in graceful arcs and curves around obstacles, and sometimes in confusing swirls and spirals.

Metaphors for chi movement can be seen in nature. For example, a fallen tree will sometimes land in a stream, causing an obstruction. Most of the water finds a way to flow around it. But some backs up behind the tree, becoming trapped in an eddy. If the tree is not moved, the water in the eddy eventually stagnates. Chi behaves in much the same way. It is important to keep chi in motion, flowing freely without encumbrance.

Feng shui philosophy centers on the observable benefits derived from the correct placement of human-made structures—including roofs, walls, doorways, and furnishings—so that chi pathways remain open.

Chinese refer to the unfettered movement of chi balanced with both yin and yang as "the cosmic breath of the dragon" (or sheng chi). This creates a desirable environment of vibrant energy that promotes mental, physical, and spiritual health.

Chi caught in a deep windowless corner of a house or in a stuffy, enclosed room, begins to sour or turn foul. Its flow clogs up and, like water, its vital force swirls into an eddy of confusion. In traditional feng shui, this stale energy is called "the killing breath" (or shar chi).

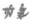

The people of China understand the divine interplay of heaven and earth energies, and allow it to govern their daily lives. They consult feng shui masters for guidance in every activity, in making crucial decisions, planning momentous events, even in the simple act of where to place a new piece of furniture in a room. Good luck, good fortune, and good health are directly related to the harmonious balancing of yin and yang, and the unobstructed flow of beneficial sheng chi.

Our environment affects our moods in subtle, but profound ways. Many of my students tell me that when they are sad or depressed (yin emotions), they take a walk outdoors under the open sky to absorb yang energy to balance the yin. The desire to bring the yin and yang into harmony is intuitive. Our entire being naturally aspires to maintaining the equilibrium.

With conscious effort and an understanding of chi dynamics, it is possible to identify chi flow problems quickly and correct them. In this way, we keep a healthy balance of yin/yang, and invite the dragon's cosmic breath to mingle with our own.

Adjusting to the Chi in Nature

I instruct my students to take advantage, whenever possible, of the chi found in nature. To do this, we need to consider the profound effects of the gravitational pull of the moon, the magnetic strength of the north and south poles, and the tremendous solar power of the sun. The chi generated by these elements magnifies the benefits of the chi kung exercises presented in this book.

I recommend using these general guidelines (in the Northern Hemisphere) to intensify the influence of the sun and magnetic poles in daily workouts:

Time of Day	Best Direction to Face
Early Morning	East
Mid-day and afternoon	South
Evening and night	North

• In the early morning, do your healing, chi kung movements facing the rising sun. Fresh yang energy will invigorate you after a night of yin sleep.

• If you do chi kung during the mid-day or afternoon, face the south. The fire energy coming from this direction stimulates expansion of the mind. This is a good thing to do in the middle of your work day.

• In the evening, after the powerful sun sets, do the exercises facing north. From here we receive the flow of yin, the fluid energy of water, like a trickling stream, or bubbling spring. This energy induces calm after a day of hectic activity.

Each direction at different times of the day encourages the unobstructed flow of energies to penetrate your meridians. Following these guidelines will help capture the healing influence of nature's power, and make the exercises more effective.

Like phototropic plants that daily lean toward the life-giving sunlight, we are intuitively attracted to health. If it is difficult for you to follow the guidelines and face the recommended direction at a certain time of day, find an area in your home or workplace where the energy enlivens you. Some people prefer natural settings, like a park or a backyard. Others feel more comfortable in the solitude of their bedrooms. Pay attention to your surroundings, and how they make you feel. Find a spot where you are peaceful and happy, reflective and alive. When you select the location for your daily workout, quietly look around. If you are in a room, take note of light sources and where the furniture is placed. Move things around, and make the room yours. If you are outside, look at the shapes and colors of the trees, where the flowerbeds are, and notice the direction of the wind. You can instinctively locate the best place to be, where chi energy flows most freely.

Feng shui demands that you incorporate an "Awareness Factor" into your life—be conscious of your surroundings, observe the details of your environment, and feel the energy as it flows to you.

Using Chi to Heal the Internal Body

Each of us generates a type of energy called jung chi, which radiates from us, and forms a pulsating energy field that encircles our bodies. When we are happy, our chi vibrates at a high frequency, and people around us feel our joy. When we are sad, people feel our sorrow, and are affected by the yin chi we emit.

Our chi weakens or strengthens under the influence of many things—the weather, our environment, our diets, our thoughts. There is always the potential to upset the equilibrium of chi in our bodies, creating too much yin, too much yang, or blocks in our meridians and channels.

When the dynamics of our lives cause mood swings, self-inflicted stress, and negative thought, we create an imbalance. These conditions change the flow of our chi, and cause a cycle that eventually manifests as illness. For example, when we are angry, our fists and jaw clench, our shoulders and stomach tighten, and our hearts pound. These tight bundles of emotion are like fallen trees in the meridian stream (energy channel) of our internal organs. Chi flow is blocked, and although it will move around the tensed area, some chi will be caught in an eddy, and begin to stagnate.

Meridian blocks are subtle. It is difficult to feel the obstructions. We may feel a little pent-up, uncomfortable, or irritated by nagging little pains. But we tend to push on, stressing, anguishing, and creating more blocks. If the meridians are not cleared, the cells they nourish start to weaken, eventually causing organs to malfunction, and cells to mutate. It is only when illness strikes that we begin to seek help.

Chi kung, exercises used for healing, have been proven through the centuries to clear the meridian blocks of obstructions, and generate the healthy flow of chi.

In traditional feng shui, if a master finds sharp angles affecting the streams of energy around a house, he suggests planting a tree to soften the angle to give the chi a rounded form to navigate past the energy trap. Chi kung uses a combination of dan tien (vertical) breathing and movement to internally massage the organs and remove meridian obstructions.

Each exercise is designed to target specific parts of the body, and free the systemic flow of chi. The gentle twisting of the torso, the rise and fall of the arms and hands, and the rotation of the spine and hips invigorate the muscles and organs with chi. The body awakens as the "cosmic breath of the dragon" courses through the meridians and into the cells.

Proper breathing is vitally important. It brings life-giving chi into the body. The deep, abdominal expansion of each breath gently stimulates the organs, pressing them against each other in a mild massage.

This breathing technique, combined with chi kung movements, elongates and adjusts the meridians to dislodge obstructions. The healing components of chi kung exercise and proper breathing take in the chi from our earth and sky, balance the yin and yang energies in the body, stimulate the internal organs, gently flex and stretch the muscles, and open the channels to allow the body's natural healing powers to work.

The First 16 Secrets of Chi

T he human body, like any growing thing, has an automatic incli-
nation for the equilibrium of health. It instinctually moves toward
life and the abundant life-sustaining elements in nature. Illness and
injury occur when some part of the body falls out of balance.

For years, we've been told that physical exercise is the best method
of keeping fit and living a long and healthy life. But most of today's
fitness regimes include vigorous movements that mirror the hectic
stresses levied on our everyday activities. These popular forms of
exercise promise ebullient health, but do little to release the tension
and strain our psyches and bodies endure during the course of a day.
Instead, they hammer at our joints and muscles, making it difficult to
sustain any type of program consistency. We become so worn down
that all too often we neglect even simple physical activities, like walking and stretching.

I call the exercises in this chapter "the first sixteen secrets of chi."
They are the foundation of the t'ai chi internal healing discipline,
chi kung, and are the most powerful movements ever devised by man.
These ancient techniques for correct posture and breathing were
designed to open energetic pathways within the body. Each movement, one position flowing into the next, carries a profound, hidden
secret.

Little children know that a secret—a whispered message of hidden wisdom packed with valuable information—is shared with a
special friend. The exercises in this book unlock the secrets your body
has been waiting to tell you, clues to its longevity and perfect health.

You must listen in a very special way: not with your ears, for the
flow of chi is much too subtle to vibrate the eardrum; and not with

your heart, for its constant beat will drown the delicate whispers of chi flow. Your body will talk to you through the shiver and tingle of every nerve and sinew, as they vibrate with the light of healing energy.

Feng Shui Guidelines

Location. Part of the feng shui notion with regard to chi exercise is the positioning of your body relative to earth and sky, trees (any plants), walls (mountains), and water.

Wherever you do your exercises, be sure you are centered. Have solid footing for any standing exercise. You might even be in the shower, an ideal location for many chi kung movements, with warm, clear water running over your shoulders, and a flat, traction-secure plane beneath your feet. Or you may be outside, or on a gym floor sharing your space with other students. Be careful to balance your stance. Keep enough room around you to move unimpeded, so that the field of your chi opens most favorably to the ambient chi.

Mirrors are useful. One student told me that she exercises in front of a full-length mirror because her body teaches her by its posture how to move. Mirrors add depth to a room, complementing the yang energy of the sky.

This student also said she sometimes does her workout in a dark room or with her eyes closed so she may concentrate on how her body feels. This way she can "see" the universal energy surging through her like waves filled with sunlight. Such darkness promotes yin.

Locating the ideal place for your workout will depend on whether yang or yin energy dominates your chi at that particular moment. Follow your own jung chi (chi your body generates). You will be able to feel the subtle energy of a place, and if it is right for you, your jung chi will resonate, and you'll feel comfortable in the area.

Earth and sky. No matter where you stand, imagine the curve of the earth below you. If you are on the ground, in a house, or high up in a skyscraper, imagine your bare feet touching the substance—the rock and soil—of our planet beneath you. Send your toes and heels like roots downward to anchor yourself. Extend your neck as high as it will go, lifting your head into the heavens. Stand or sit tall, back straight. Imagine the arc of the sky like a crest above your head. Support the sky with the uppermost curve of your skull.

Between the parallel arcs of earth and sky, you are in the middle of a rainbow that circles the planet like a halo. Notice the colors. Above you is the sunny, bright red and orange sky. And below is the green-to-blue-to purple of earth and sea. Imagine your body blending with the rainbow, growing upward and downward into it.

If there is a ceiling above, pretend it isn't there. Only the sky exists.

Trees. Whatever house plants you have, or the trees and shrubbery around you, any growing and flowering vegetation tends to curve yang energy. Consider the effect these plants have on the light in the air. Circles of chi will radiate from the plants.

Position yourself near or far from the plants, according to the concentration of their life force and the effect it has on you.

Walls. Vertical or ascending surfaces block or channel chi. Be sure to face the breaks in walls, hills, and mountains: openings like windows or valleys that allow air and light and distance to accelerate toward you.

Water. The ocean is the most potent medium of yin water power. At some point during your workout, turn to face a water source: a faucet, fountain, stream, or lake. Maybe there's a window looking out upon the rain. When your sweat flows you might have to turn away from the water and begin to cool down, or splash into it for the same reason.

Once you have completed your exercises you must apply water to your skin either by washing your hands and face (try the "Cat Washing Face" form of "Tiger Eyes" below, but with wet hands instead of dry) or by bathing.

General Guidelines

Dan tien or **vertical breathing** is the ancient technique of inhaling and exhaling air (and chi) to expand the diaphragm. Pressure from the distended diaphragm pushes against the organs and muscles of the lower abdomen, causing it to swell, then flatten with each complete breath. This movement gently massages the vital organs, and creates beneficial feng shui as your internal landscape is lifted and lowered to allow chi to freely circulate through the area.

If you ever wondered about the symbolism of Buddha's round belly, it is this: he reminds us where the chi is. Buddha is not plump or fat. His belly is filled with chi. If you rub his tummy, you receive good luck from his chi center.

When you breathe in, think of the happy Buddha, and inflate the balloon of your belly. This area is shaped like a circle, with the upper part along the rib cage, and the lower section cupped by the pelvis. This circle represents the source of chi in your body. Its center is the navel.

Always inhale and exhale through your nose. Your nostrils are lined with hair that act as a natural filter to clarify the air.

Your chest should remain still during this entire process, while the balloon of your abdomen, your dan tien, inflates and deflates. It is sometimes a good idea to monitor your technique by placing one hand on your chest, and the other on your dan tien. There should be no movement in the chest area, while the abdomen expands or deflates.

It is important to remember: do not hold your breath while practicing this technique. The flow of air should follow your natural breathing rhythm. Sometime people feel a little dizzy the first couple of times they try this new way of breathing. For most of our lives we use our lungs, taking in shallow breaths. Dan tien breathing brings much more oxygen into the body, and the untrained practitioner may experience mild hyperventilation. Don't be alarmed. If this happens, relax. Stop the dan tien breathing, and breathe normally, through your upper chest. When you are comfortable, begin vertical breathing again.

When performing the exercises, position yourself in the prescribed starting posture. Inhale. Always begin the movements of the exercises with an inhalation.

We also recommend that you place your tongue lightly against you upper palate to ensure that your juices continue to flow in your mouth. It is much easier to perform this type of breathing when the muscles of your mouth are relaxed. The tongue in this position will assist you.

Note: please remember to perform vertical breathing throughout all of the following exercises.

The Chi "Ball." In many of the following exercises you are asked to visualize lifting and moving an imaginary ball of chi energy. The size of this sphere of healing light will vary, depending on the shape of your hands.

Once you curl your fingers, a chi ball will instantly appear where you imagine it. Some people have a difficult time "seeing" a visualization. This is not important when working with chi. With a little practice, you will feel the energy's heat penetrating your hands from the palms to the tips of your fingers.

The posture. For each of the 16 exercises, you must first literally set yourself straight, in a balanced pose that places the least strain on all your bones, joints, organs, and extremities. Most of the exercises can be done in a standing or seated position.

Standing position. Place your feet shoulder-width apart. The spacing should allow you to make two fists joined together between your knees.

Stand upright and tall, and look at your left foot. Turn the toes inward very slightly. Imagine a line running from the outside crescent of your little toe to the outer tip of your right shoulder. Do the same with your right foot and left shoulder. The triangles made by these two intersecting lines will meet (at the crossing of the X) in the bottom half of the abdomen. The deep breath you inhale should reach this point, the center of the X.

Square yourself. Imagine a board in a straight line across your shoulders. The X supports this board and makes it level and strong.

Seated Position. Move your buttocks to the edge of your chair. Sit upright, as tall and straight as you can. Keep feet flat on the floor or ground. Even in a sitting position you can imagine an X shape rising from the outside of your little toes, crossing through the abdomen, and ending at the outer tips of your squared shoulders.

Your hands. During the exercises, watch the movement of your hands. Fingers and thumb, palms and wrists are power centers for chi. Not only will your hands help shape the chi balls and direct the chi inside you, they are capable of healing by touch.

Whenever we hurt ourselves, we automatically place our hands on the afflicted area. This tells the injured tissues that the mind is paying attention. Our hands become warm, sometimes hot, as healing energy is funneled toward the pain. Our hands are the conduits of jung chi. As we hold or rub the area, the pain becomes easier to control.

While performing the different exercises, keep in mind the healing powers generated through your hands. They are designed to increase the already powerful healing force that is naturally available to you.

Exercises for special needs. Just as a doctor prescribes medicines for certain ailments, Chinese practitioners of chi have told their patients to do specific exercises to restore their organs, joints, and muscles. Each of the exercises in this chapter provides regenerative energy to parts of your body. You should perform them all, in the order they are presented. The sixteen exercises complement each other and target the entire body.

If you are suffering from a health problem, find it on the chart below. Make a mental note of the exercise (or exercises) that addresses the problem. Do the entire "16 secrets" program, and sometime during the day (when you think of it) take a little extra time to do the exercise that targets your specific area of concern.

Allergies
Exercise 1: Rowing the Boat

Alzheimer's disease
Exercise 1: Rowing the Boat
Exercise 2: Awakening the Giant
Exercise 9: Balancing the Earth

Ankles
Exercise 6: Crane Walking in the Clouds
Exercise 14: Secret Fountain of Youth

Arthritis
Exercise 1: Rowing the Boat
Exercise 4: Rocking the Ocean
Exercise 6: Crane Walking in the Clouds
Exercise 7: Rounding the Heaven and Earth Energy
Exercise 8: Turning Over the Earth and Supporting the Sky
Exercise 9: Balancing the Earth
Exercise 11: Eagle Looking for Food
Exercise 14: Secret Fountain of Youth
Exercise 15: Crane Form: Bending Knees on Floor

Asthma
Exercise 1: Rowing the Boat
Exercise 13: Crane Catching the Fish
Exercise 14: Secret Fountain of Youth

Back (spinal column)
Exercise 1: Rowing the Boat
Exercise 4: Rocking the Ocean
Exercise 5: Monkey Form: Waist Turning
Exercise 9: Balancing the Earth
Exercise 11: Eagle Looking for Food
Exercise 12: Cross Hands in Front of Face
Exercise 13: Crane Catching the Fish
Exercise 15: Crane Form: Bending Knees on Floor

Balance (equilibrium)
Exercise 8: Turning Over the Earth and Supporting the Sky with Both Arms

Blood pressure
Exercise 1: Rowing the Boat
Exercise 6: Crane Walking in the Clouds

Breast cancer
Exercise 7: Rounding the Heaven and Earth Energy

Circulatory system (blood pressure and general blood circulation)
Exercise 1: Rowing the Boat
Exercise 6: Crane Walking in the Clouds
Exercise 8: Turning Over the Earth and Supporting the Sky with Both Arms
Exercise 14: Secret Fountain of Youth

Cognitive powers
Exercise 3: Hang Loose

Diabetes
Exercise 1: Rowing the Boat
Exercise 8: Turning Over the Earth and Supporting the Sky with Both Arms

Exercise 10: Tiger Eyes
Exercise 14: Secret Fountain of Youth

Digestion
Exercise 3: Hang Loose
Exercise 13: Crane Catching the Fish
Exercise 14: Secret Fountain of Youth

Drowsiness
Exercise 10: Tiger Eyes

Ear (inner ear)
Exercise 8: Turning Over the Earth and Supporting the Sky with Both Arms

Endocrine system (thyroid, pituitary gland, hormone regulation)
Exercise 4: Rocking the Ocean
Exercise 6: Crane Walking in the Clouds
Exercise 7: Rounding the Heaven and Earth Energy
Exercise 12: Cross Hands in Front of Face
Exercise 13: Crane Catching the Fish
Exercise 14: Secret Fountain of Youth

Eyes (nearsightedness, farsightedness)
Exercise 10: Tiger Eyes

Face (wrinkles)
Exercise 10: Tiger Eyes
Exercise 11: Eagle Looking for Food

Face (natural facelift)
Exercise 11: Eagle Looking for Food

Flu symptoms
Exercise 9: Balancing the Earth

Exercise 14: Secret Fountain of Youth

Gums
Exercise 11: Eagle Looking for Food
Headache (migraine)
Exercise 9: Balancing the Earth

Heart problems
Exercise 1: Rowing the Boat
Exercise 2: Awakening the Giant
Exercise 7: Rounding the Heaven and Earth Energy

Immune system
Exercise 14: Secret Fountain of Youth

Joints
Exercise 6: Crane Walking in the Clouds
Exercise 11: Eagle Looking for Food
Exercise 14: Secret Fountain of Youth
Exercise 15: Crane Form: Bending Knees on Floor

Kidneys
Exercise 5: Monkey Form: Waist Turning

Knees
Exercise 6: Crane Walking in the Clouds

Liver
Exercise 2: Awakening the Giant

Lung (congestion, shortness of breath)
Exercise 2: Awakening the Giant
Exercise 7: Rounding the Heaven and Earth Energy
Exercise 13: Crane Catching the Fish
Exercise 14: Secret Fountain of Youth

Memory
Exercise 1: Rowing the Boat
Exercise 2: Awakening the Giant

Menstrual cramps
Exercise 4: Rocking the Ocean
Exercise 12: Cross Hands in Front of Face
Exercise 13: Crane Catching the Fish

Neck
Exercise 9: Balancing the Earth

Nervous system
Exercise 1: Rowing the Boat
Exercise 14: Secret Fountain of Youth

Osteosclerosis
Exercise 4: Rocking the Ocean
Exercise 7: Rounding the Heaven and Earth Energy
Exercise 14: Secret Fountain of Youth
Exercise 15: Crane Form: Bending Knees on Floor

Parkinson's disease
Exercise 2: Awakening the Giant
Exercise 9: Balancing the Earth
Exercise 14: Secret Fountain of Youth

Respiratory system
Exercise 1: Rowing the Boat
Exercise 8: Turning Over the Earth and Supporting the Sky
Exercise 13: Crane Catching the Fish
Exercise 14: Secret Fountain of Youth

Rheumatism
Exercise 7: Rounding the Heaven and Earth Energy

Exercise 11: Eagle Looking for Food
Exercise 12: Cross Hands in Front of Face
Exercise 13: Crane Catching the Fish
Exercise 14: Secret Fountain of Youth
Exercise 15: Crane Form: Bending Knees on Floor

•

Saliva
Exercise 11: Eagle Looking for Food

Sinus
Exercise 1: Rowing the Boat
Exercise 13: Crane Catching the Fish
Exercise 14: Secret Fountain of Youth

Spleen (blood filtering and low white blood cell count)
Exercise 2: Awakening the Giant

Stroke
Exercise 2: Awakening the Giant
Exercise 3: Hang Loose
Exercise 6: Crane Walking in the Clouds
Exercise 9: Balancing the Earth
Exercise 11: Eagle Looking for Food
Exercise 14: Secret Fountain of Youth

Stomach (nausea and stomach aches)
Exercise 2: Awakening the Giant
Exercise 3: Hang Loose
Exercise 13: Crane Catching the Fish
Exercise 14: Secret Fountain of Youth

Shoulder pain
Exercise 2: Awakening the Giant
Exercise 7: Rounding the Heaven and Earth Energy

Thyroid
Exercise 11: Eagle Looking for Food

Ulcers
Exercise 3: Hang Loose

Weight gain
Exercise 4: Rocking the Ocean
Exercise 5: Monkey Form: Waist Turning
Exercise 6: Crane Walking in the Clouds
Exercise 12: Cross Hands in Front of Face
Exercise 15: Crane Form: Bending Knees on Floor

Exercises for Health
and Longevity

Exercise 1

Rowing the Boat

██

The name of this exercise provides the images for correct execution of the movements. Imagine that you are in a magic boat, and you are rowing to a distant shore. Beneath the purple dream water swims a school of crystal fish. You row along, with the fish to guide you.

The exercise begins with correct dan tien breathing, gently rocking your internal organs with muscular massage. This is in preparation for the rest of the exercises.

The next series mimics the forward and back rocking movements of rowing a boat. Instead of your arms dictating the momentum of the body, your legs bend and stretch, leaning the torso toward and away from the bow of your boat.

The final phase of the exercise incorporates the arms, a pushing and pulling of imaginary oars.

Keep the image of rowing a boat in mind throughout the exercise, and create a balance between each motion and correct dan tien breathing.

██

This exercise helps in the treatment of allergies, asthma, arthritis, back pain, diabetes, and sinus problems, and it strengthens the respiratory, circulatory, and nervous systems, with particular benefit to the heart.

██

1-A

Rowing the Boat (with Your Breath)

This is the chi name for **vertical breathing,** the dan tien breathing technique. The exercise sucks oxygen into your lungs to reach the deepest and narrowest airways. It replaces the stale air that has collected there through a lifetime of shallow breaths. Therefore, it increases lung capacity. More oxygen is available for consumption, and blood circulation accelerates.

If you experience any dizziness or lightheadedness, stop the dan tien breathing, taking shallow lung-breaths, until you feel like you can begin dan tien breathing again.

NOTE: You can do this exercise standing, sitting, or lying down.

Step 1: STARTING POSITION: Place feet shoulder-width distance apart. Close your eyes.

Step 2: Put one hand on your chest.

Step 3: The other hand over your abdomen, 3 finger-widths below your navel.

Step 4: Rest your tongue against the roof of your mouth. This stimulates the glands to promote saliva, and encourages the flow of your body fluids. With all vertical breathing your tongue should be in this position.

Step 5: Inhale through the nose, taking the air all the way down into your abdomen, which will expand like an inflating balloon.

Step 6: Exhale to release the air through your nose. As you do so, imagine your body is a boat being rowed, the oars moving with your breath.

Step 7: Repeat steps 1 to 6 at least 11 times. You are on your way.

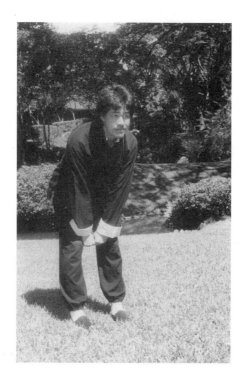

I-B

Rowing the Boat (Step Movement)

Do standing on your own or with a chair, for support.

Step 1: STARTING POSITION: Place feet shoulder-width distance apart. If standing, make two fists with your hands and place them between your knees. This will provide the proper distance between your legs.

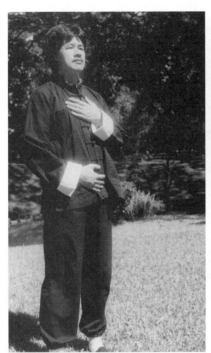
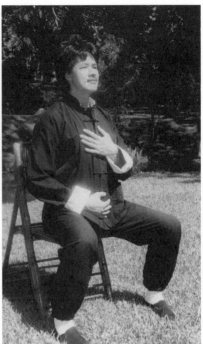

1-B

Rowing the Boat (Step Movement)

Step 2: One hand on chest.

Step 3: The other hand over your abdomen, 3 finger-widths below your navel. (If you are using your hands to support yourself with a chair, skip steps 2 and 3.) Inhale and exhale, using dan tien breathing.

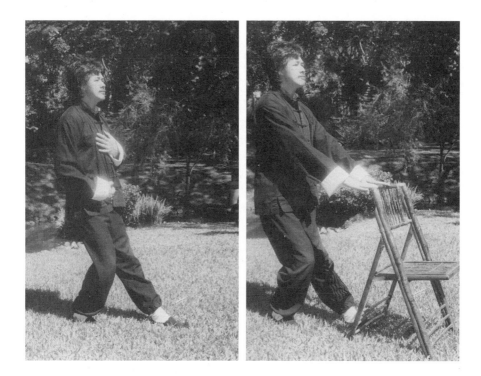

I-B

Rowing the Boat (Step Movement)

Step 4: Place one foot forward and bend the back knee, allowing body weight to rest on the back foot. (Inhale.)

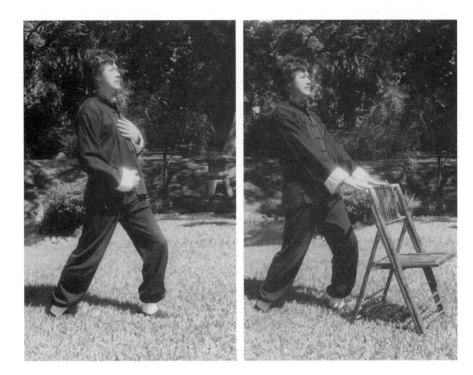

1-B

Rowing the Boat (Step Movement)

Step 5: Gently shift your body weight forward into a slight lunge—knees bent comfortably to balance the shifting of your weight. (Exhale.)

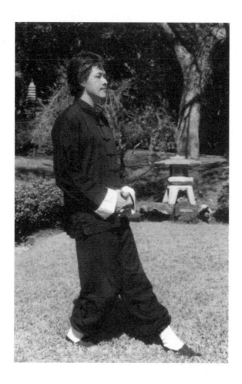

I-B

Rowing the Boat (Step Movement)

Step 6: Now shift the weight back as in step number 4. (Inhale.)

Step 7: Repeat steps 4 and 5 at least 11 times, rocking yourself forward and back.

Step 8: Now change position so your other foot is forward, and repeat the exercise. Perform vertical breathing throughout. Keep movements slow and controlled.

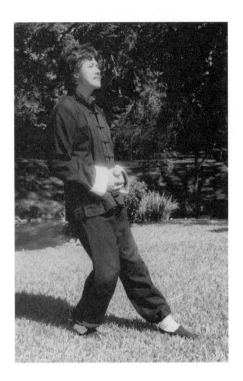

1-C

Rowing the Boat (to the Nearest Shore)

Step 1: STARTING POSITION: Standing with back erect and shoulders square, one foot forward, resting body weight on the back foot. Place both hands on your abdomen, one over the other, 3 finger-widths below your navel. (Inhale.)

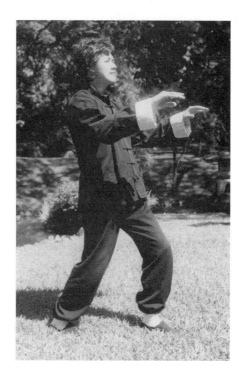

I-C

Rowing the Boat (to the Nearest Shore)

Step 2: Exhale and shift your weight forward while parting and lifting both hands forward and upward until they reach shoulder height. Do not straighten your arms all the way; keep your elbows slightly bent, palms down to collect the yin chi from Mother Earth.

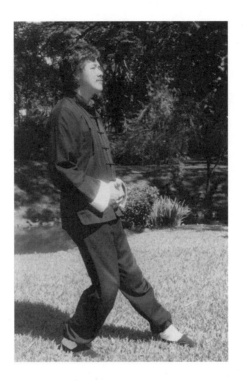

1-C

Rowing the Boat (to the Nearest Shore)

Step 3: Inhale as you shift your weight back and return your hands to your abdomen, left over right.

Repeat this movement at least 11 times, rocking yourself forward and back.

Keep your upper body vertical (perpendicular to the Earth) through the entire exercise.

Now place the other foot forward, reversing hands, and repeat the exercise. Perform vertical breathing throughout. Keep movements slow and controlled.

Exercise 2

Awakening the Giant (Memory Form)

This exercise awakens your immense power and strength, the giant that lies sleeping within your physical frame. You are asked to reach to the sky, lengthening your body, imitating the posture and grandeur of a giant.

Elongate your spine, lengthen your neck, and reach your head toward the sky. Your journey began by rowing a boat through the dream sea toward the mythical land of health and wellness, flexibility and strength. You are huge in this new land.

In our journey toward optimum health of body and mind, we are often asked to stretch beyond our normal stature, to assume a giant's strength to continue the journey. Stand as tall and broad as you can, expanding your chi to flow through your extended posture. There are no mountains (emotional or physical) that can not be conquered by your giant within.

With this exercise, the giant has awakened.

This exercise improves circulation to the brain, and enhances memory. It helps in the treatment of arthritis, Alzheimer's disease, and Parkinson's disease, and strengthens the heart, liver, lungs, spleen, and stomach. It helps prevent stroke and assists in recovery from stroke, and particularly relieves shoulder pain and stiffness.

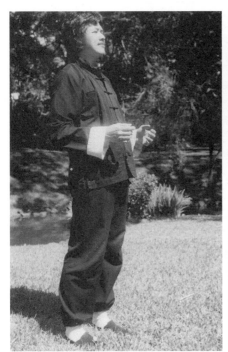 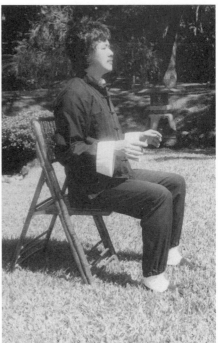

2-A

Awakening the Giant (Awakening State of Mind)

This is a "Memory Form" exercise that clears a mental path, and opens the mind to focus and concentration. Breathe through your nose, performing dan tien breathing throughout the exercise. With each inhalation, gather chi into your abdomen. Imagine the chi heating up your hands as you perform this exercise. As you exhale, shoot the chi out through your palms.

Step 1: STARTING POSITION: Sitting or standing, place feet shoulder-width distance apart, toes pointed slightly inwards. Keep elbows close to your body, bent at a 90° angle. Your hands should be relaxed, palms facing inward. Pull arms backward, keeping lower arm parallel to the ground. (Inhale.)

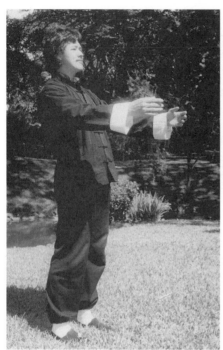 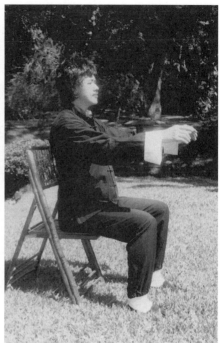

2-A

Awakening the Giant (Awakening State of Mind)

Step 2: Extend your arms forward, hands straight out in front of you. Keep elbows slightly bent, palms facing each other. (Exhale.)

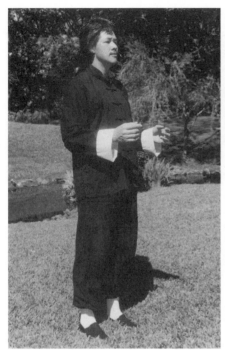
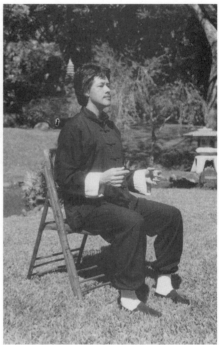

2-A

Awakening the Giant (Awakening State of Mind)

Step 3: Bring the hands back into position 1. (Inhale.)

Repeat this "In & Out" movement at least 11 times. Perform vertical breathing throughout. Keep movements slow and controlled.

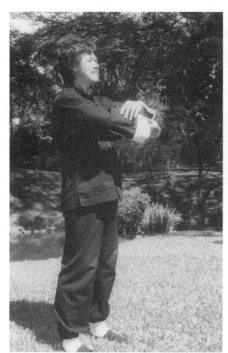
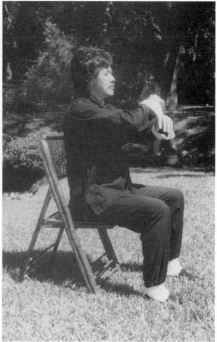

2-B

Awakening the Giant (Spreading the Path)

This is the second "Memory Form." It opens the path further for the giant by gathering chi into the heart and pumping oxygenated chi back into the air before you.

Step 1: STARTING POSITION: Stand or sit tall, feet shoulder-width distance apart, toes pointed slightly inward. Cross your arms loosely in front of your chest, palms facing down. (Inhale.)

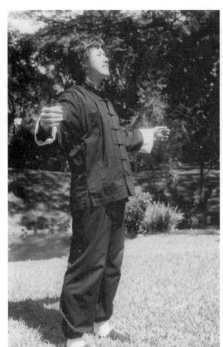 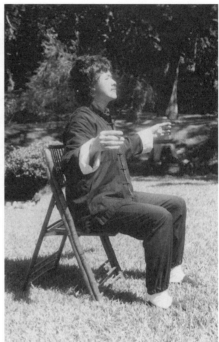

2-B

Awakening the Giant (Spreading the Path)

Step 2: Open your arms, expanding the chest like a bird in flight. (Exhale.)

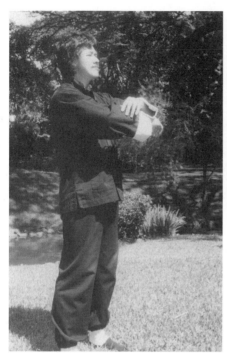
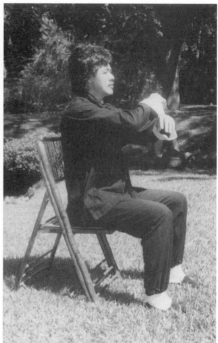

2-B

Awakening the Giant (Spreading the Path)

Step 3: Return arms to starting position. (Inhale.)

Repeat Steps 1 through 3 at least 11 times. Do vertical breathing throughout. Keep movements slow and controlled.

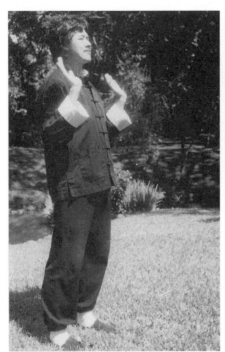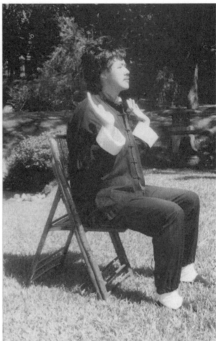

2-C

Awakening the Giant (Enlightened by Heaven)

Step 1: STARTING POSITION: Stand or sit tall, feet shoulder-width distance apart, toes pointed inward slightly. Raise arms to shoulder-height. Flex wrists so that your palms are facing the heavens to collect the strong yang energy of the sky. (Inhale.)

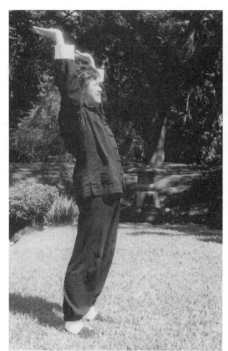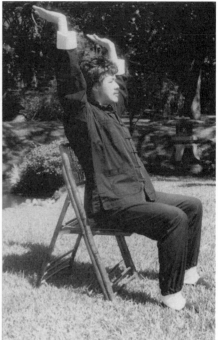

2-C

Awakening the Giant (Enlightened by Heaven)

Step 2: Balancing an imaginary chi ball in the palm of each hand, extend arms high overhead, to a point where your slightly bent elbows are just behind your ears. Press palms toward the sky. (Exhale.)

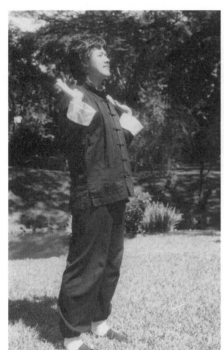
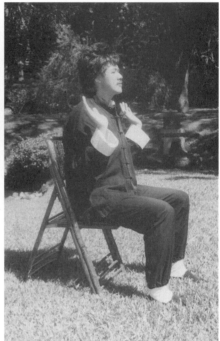

2-C

Awakening the Giant (Enlightened by Heaven)

Step 3: Return arms to starting position. (Inhale.)

Repeat Steps 1 through 3 at least 11 times. Do vertical breathing throughout. Keep movements slow and controlled.

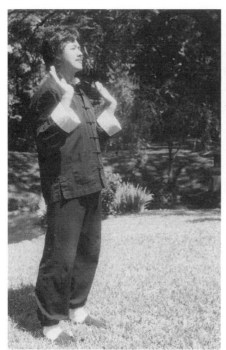
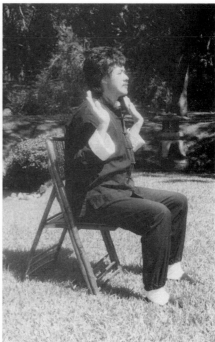

2-D

Awakening the Giant (Holding on to the Path)

Step 1: STARTING POSITION: Stand or sit tall, feet shoulder-width distance apart, toes pointed slightly inward. Raise arms to just below shoulder-height. Wrists flexed with palms slightly forward. (Inhale.)

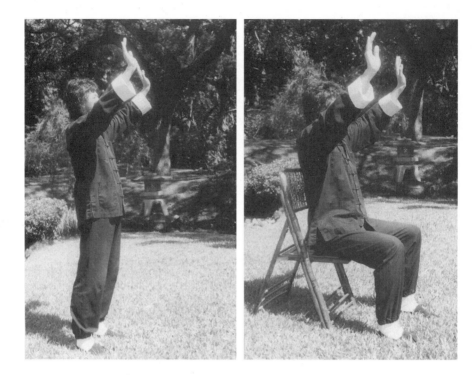

2-D

Awakening the Giant (Holding on to the Path)

Step 2: Press palms upward as if pushing a chi ball in each hand. Arms should be extended in front of the head. (Exhale.)

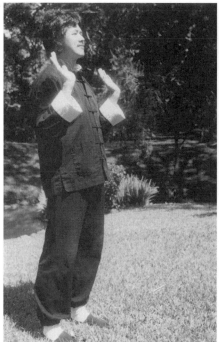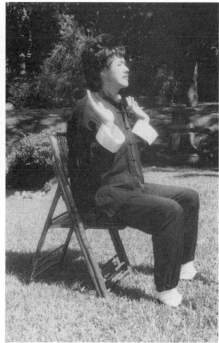

2-D

Awakening the Giant (Holding on to the Path)

Step 3: Return arms to starting position. (Inhale.)

Repeat Steps 1 through 3 at least 11 times. Do vertical breathing throughout. Keep movements slow and controlled.

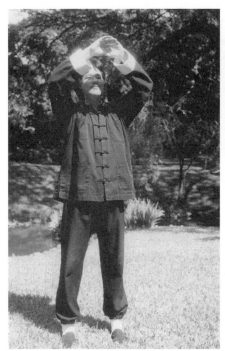 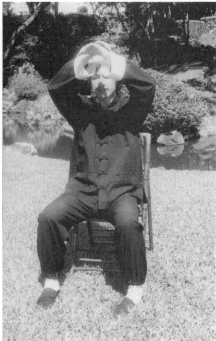

2-E

Awakening the Giant (Embrace the Universe)

Step 1: STARTING POSITION: Stand or sit tall, feet shoulder-width distance apart, toes pointed slightly inward. Cross your hands in front of your forehead, palms facing outward. (Inhale.)

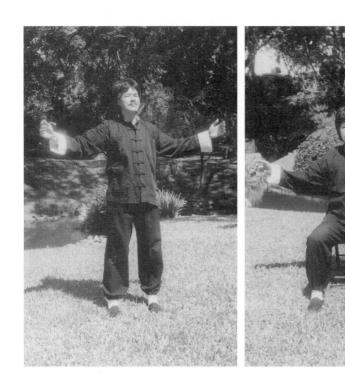

2-E

Awakening the Giant (Embrace the Universe)

Step 2: Open your arms, palms forward, as if welcoming a friend into your home. (Exhale.)

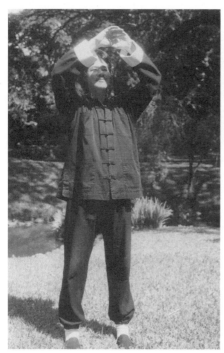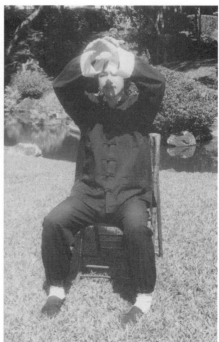

2-E

Awakening the Giant (Embrace the Universe)

Step 3: Return to starting position. (Inhale.)

Repeat Steps 1 through 3 at least 11 times, alternately crossing left over right and right over left. Remember to continue vertical breathing throughout. Keep movements slow and controlled.

Exercise 3

Hang Loose

After moving to Hawai'i, I changed the name of this exercise to "Hang Loose" from its original name, "Hands Loose." Whenever I said, "OK, we are going to do the Hands Loose exercise," people always said, "What? Hang Loose?" In the Islands, Hang Loose means to relax, calm down, enjoy the moment. I liked this, and changed the name. Really it means the same thing.

This exercise gently expands the torso, allowing "breathing space" for the stomach and digestive tract. The subtle vibrations of chi energy also stimulate an increased flow of nutrient-enriched blood to the brain to help in the prevention of strokes. Through the centuries, the Chinese have used this simple movement to treat ulcers, digestive disorders, and strokes. Recently, it has been used to offset appetite loss caused by chemotherapy treatments.

While doing this exercise, it is easy to let the momentum of the swinging arms take over the movement. Steady the momentum by controlling the lifting and lowering of your arms, as yin energy is lifting your arms from below, and yang energy is lowering them from above.

It is also important to remember that with the arms overhead it is tempting to arch your lower back. As you are doing your dan tien breathing, try to keep your back comfortably stable.

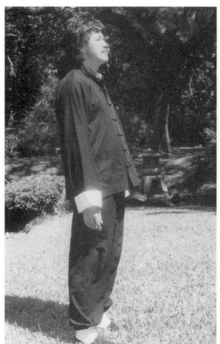 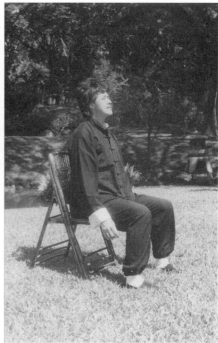

3-A

Hang Loose

Step 1: STARTING POSITION: Stand or sit with feet shoulder-width distance apart, toes pointed slightly inward. Shake your hands at your sides, relaxing your shoulders, and loosening all of the tension in the arms. (Inhale and exhale.)

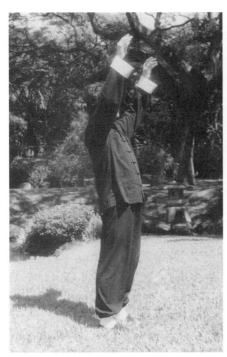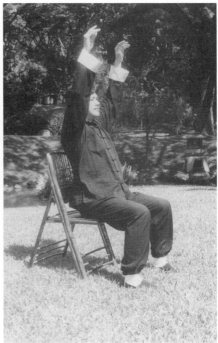

3-A

Hang Loose

Step 2: Keeping arms extended, elbows slightly bent, swing arms in front of your body and raise to overhead position. The swinging motion should be a slow creation of a broad arc. (Inhale.)

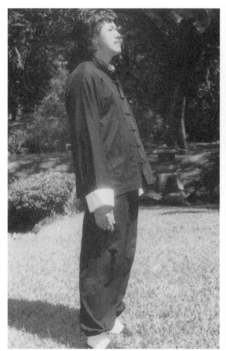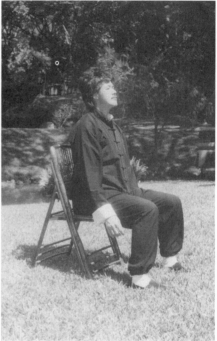

3-A
Hang Loose

Step 3: Swing the arms back down to the starting position. (Exhale.)

Repeat Steps 1 through 3 at least 11 times. Do vertical breathing throughout. Keep movements slow and controlled.

Exercise 4

Rocking the Ocean

How much force does it take to affect a body of water as massive as an ocean? The answer is—very little. Just a grain of sand dropped into a pond creates a ripple, so putting one foot into the ocean will rock the water. Small actions initiate grand effects.

In Kung Fu training, a flexible back is the center of all movement. It is also the central conduit for healing. If you can keep your back pliable, your muscles and organs—all of which are connected to the back either directly or through the central nervous system—will benefit.

This exercise is designed to make dramatic changes in the endocrine system, and can be used to release the meridian blocks that cause weight gain. It was also used in ancient times to clear the meridian blocks responsible for painful arthritis, osteoporosis, and osteosclerosis. The twisting movements stretch and relax stiffness in the torso to relieve lower back pain and menstrual cramps.

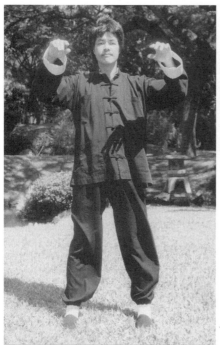 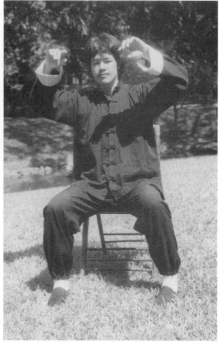

4-A

Rocking the Ocean

Step 1: STARTING POSITION: Stand or sit with feet shoulder-width distance apart, toes turned inward slightly. Lift both arms to shoulder height, elbows bent in a 90° angle, palms facing down. (Inhale and exhale.)

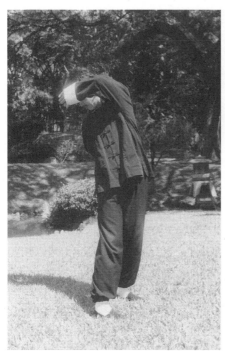
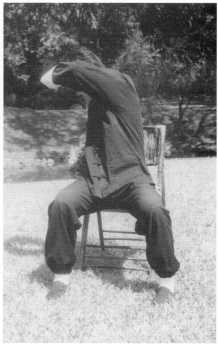

4-A

Rocking the Ocean

Step 2: Twist your torso to the right (clockwise), and move the back of your left hand toward your forehead, palm slightly cupped. Simultaneously, wrap your right arm behind you until it reaches the back plate of your left hip, palm slightly cupped. As your torso completes the twist, look down at your left heel. (Inhale)

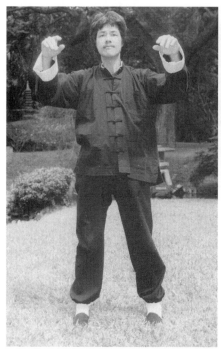 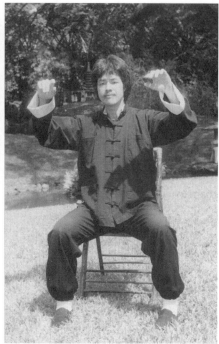

4-A

Rocking the Ocean

Step 3: Return to the starting position, facing forward, shoulders square. (Exhale.)

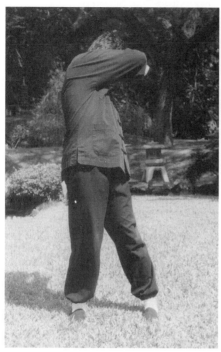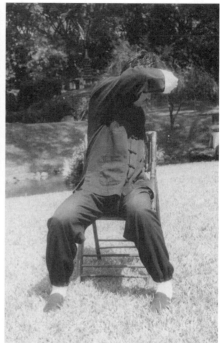

4-A

Rocking the Ocean

Step 4: Switch hands, and perform the movement with your right hand on your forehead, left hand wrapping around your back to your right hip. Twist your torso backward toward the left, and look at your right heel. (Inhale.)

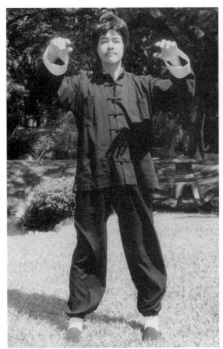 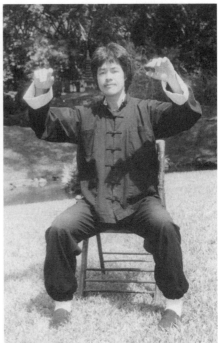

4-A

Rocking the Ocean

Step 5: END POSITION: Repeat Steps 1 through 5 at least 11 times, twisting from the right to left, alternately, and ending facing forward, elbows bent, and palms down. Do vertical breathing throughout. Keep movements slow and controlled.

Exercise 5

Monkey Form, Waist Turning

The monkey god, according to Chinese beliefs, moves with exuberant vitality and supple grace. While performing the exercises in this series, imagine yourself as a monkey and adopt its agile flexibility.

The twisting movements from extreme left to extreme right are done within one deep, complete breath (inhale and exhale). The lower back is a very narrow pivoting point. (Be sure to move slowly and smoothly to control the momentum created by the twisting of the torso.)

The spine is the primary support system in the body. The Chinese believe that if you have back pain, you have lost 90% of your natural energy. This exercise improves back flexibility, relaxes the muscles of the back, pumps vital healing energy to the kidneys, and as an added bonus, creates an internal environment that allows reduction of body weight.

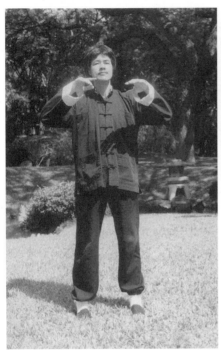 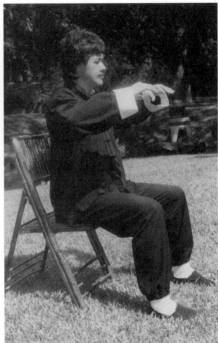

5-A
Monkey Form, Waist Turning

Step 1: STARTING POSITION: Stand or sit with feet shoulder-width distance apart, toes turned inward slightly. Lift both arms to shoulder height, elbows bent in a 30° angle, palms facing down. (Inhale and exhale.)

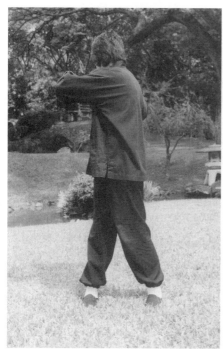 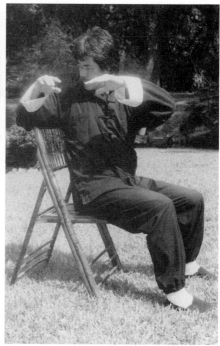

5-A

Monkey Form, Waist Turning

Step 2: Keeping feet planted, back as straight as possible, and arms still at shoulder-height, twist the torso to the right, turning as far back as possible. (Inhale.)

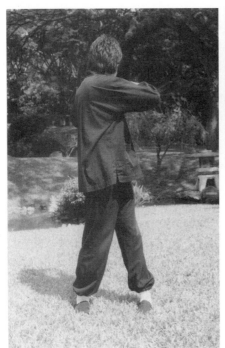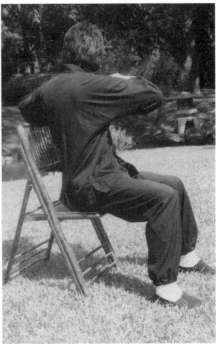

5-A

Monkey Form, Waist Turning

Step 3: Rotating past the starting position, continue to twist to the left. (Inhale.)

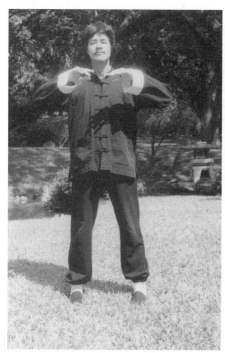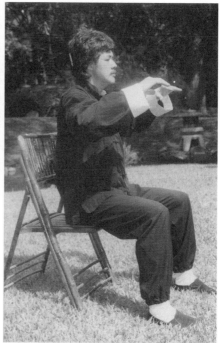

5-A

Monkey Form, Waist Turning

Step 4: END POSITION: Return to starting position, facing forward. (Exhale.)

Repeat Steps 1 through 4 at least 11 times, twisting from the right to left, alternately, and ending facing forward, elbows bent, and palms down. Do vertical breathing throughout. Each time you face forward, exhale. Each time you twist, inhale. Keep movements slow and controlled.

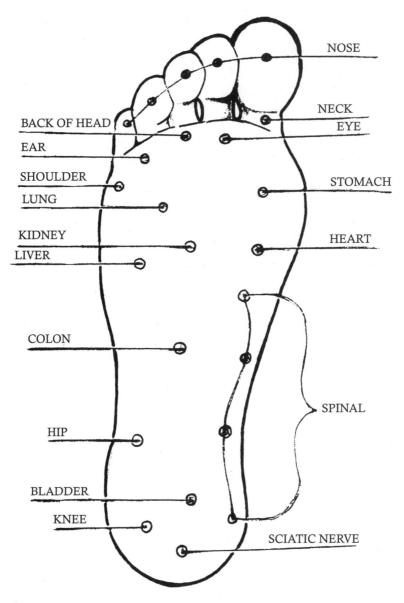

NOSE

NECK

EYE

BACK OF HEAD

EAR

SHOULDER

STOMACH

LUNG

KIDNEY

HEART

LIVER

COLON

SPINAL

HIP

BLADDER

KNEE

SCIATIC NERVE

6

Crane Walking in the Clouds (Crane Form) — Foot Diagram

Exercise 6

Crane Walking in the Clouds (Crane Form)

This Crane Form exercise is called Crane Walking in the Clouds. It's also been called Sky Walking because the movements feel as if you are stepping through fluffy mist, brushing the wisps of white vapor out of the way with the opening and closing of your hands.

It is important here, as with all of the exercises, to focus on your breathing. This is a form of acupuncture massage on the soles of the feet. When you move up to the balls of each foot, you massage the pressure points that service the nose, back of the head, ears, eyes, shoulders, lungs, stomach, kidney, liver, and heart. You also stretch and open the chi channels to the colon, hip, and spinal column. (See diagram opposite.)

When you press your hands open and closed, you send additional energy to the head area, pituitary and pineal glands, heart, liver, lungs, ears, sinuses, shoulders and arms, diaphragm, spleen, gallbladder, bladder, ovary/testicles, sacrum, coccyx, kidneys, adrenal glands, prostate/uterus, thyroid, throat, and the dual lobes of the brain. (See diagram on the next page.)

Visualize breathing through palms and feet.

This exercise relieves the pain of arthritis in the hands, back pain, inflamed or stiff finger joints, knee pain, ankle pain, and Achilles tendon pain. Because of the acupuncture massage effect of the movements, this exercise is also beneficial in getting needed healing energy to the circulatory system, and helps to prevent strokes. The twisting movements stimulate the endocrine system to counteract weight disorders.

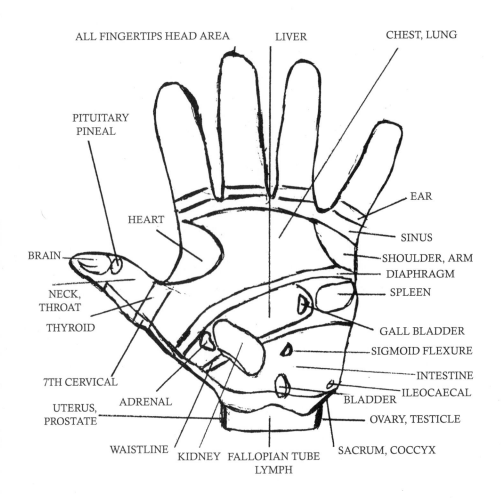

LEFT HAND PALM UP

6

Crane Walking in the Clouds (Crane Form) — Hand Diagram

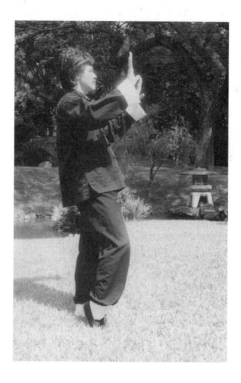

6

Crane Walking in the Clouds (Crane Form)—Standing Position

Step 1: STARTING POSITION: Stand with feet shoulder-width distance apart, toes turned inward slightly.

STANDING: Extend both arms in front of you at shoulder height. Bend elbows slightly with wrists flexed, and palms facing outward. Spread your fingers as wide as possible. Simultaneously, while spreading your fingers, lift the heel of the right foot, pressing the ball of the foot into the ground, and gently bending the right knee. Try to keep the hips level. (Inhale.)

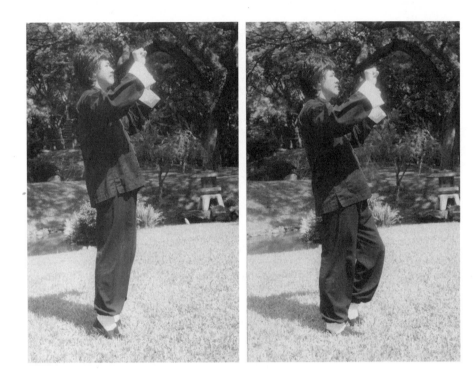

6

Crane Walking in the Clouds (Crane Form)—Standing Position

Step 2: STANDING: Elevate both heels, balancing on the balls of both feet. Close hands, making a tight fist. Exhale, and bring the right heel to the ground, leaving the left heel raised. Bend left knee slightly to keep hips level. (Exhale.)

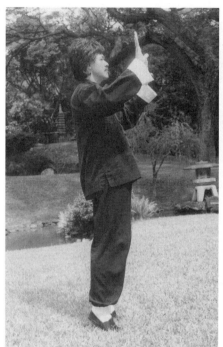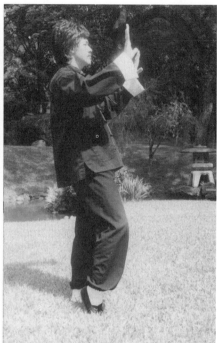

6

Crane Walking in the Clouds (Crane Form)—Standing Position

Step 3: STANDING: Elevate both heels again, balancing on the balls of both feet. Open hands, and spread fingers. Bring the left heel to the ground, leaving the right heel raised. Keep right knee bent slightly to hip level. (Inhale.)

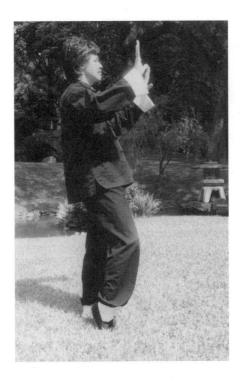

6

Crane Walking in the Clouds (Crane Form)—Standing Position

Step 4: ENDING POSITION: You are now back at the starting position.

Repeat the exercise (Steps 1 through 3) 11 times, opening and closing the hands while alternating the rise and fall of the right and left heels. Do vertical breathing throughout, remembering to always inhale with open hands.

Keep all movements slow and controlled.

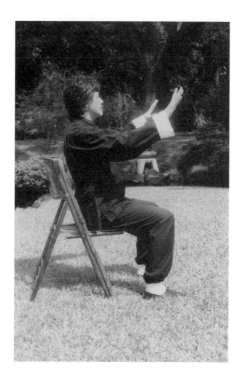

6

Crane Walking in the Clouds (Crane Form)—Sitting Position

Step 1: SITTING: Extend both arms in front of you at shoulder height. Bend elbows slightly with wrists flexed, and palms facing outward. Spread your fingers as wide as possible. Keep feet flat on the ground. (Inhale.)

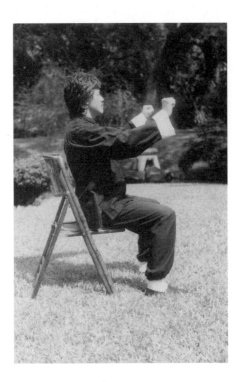

6

Crane Walking in the Clouds (Crane Form)—Sitting Position

Step 2: SITTING: Close hands, making a tight fist. Keep feet flat on the ground. (Exhale.)

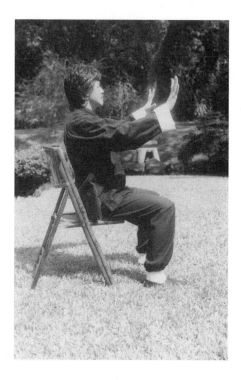

6

Crane Walking in the Clouds (Crane Form)—Sitting Position

Step 3: SITTING: Open hands, spreading fingers. Keep feet flat on the ground. (Inhale.)

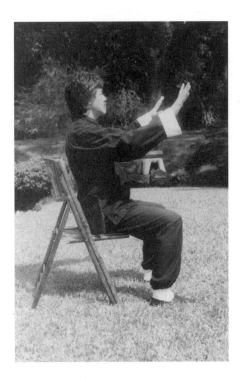

6

Crane Walking in the Clouds (Crane Form)—Sitting Position

Step 4: SITTING: You are now back at the starting position. Repeat the exercise (Steps 1 through 3) 11 times, opening and closing the hands. Do vertical breathing throughout, remembering to always inhale with open hands.

Keep all movements slow and controlled.

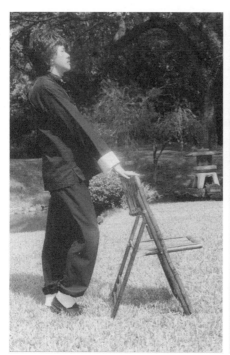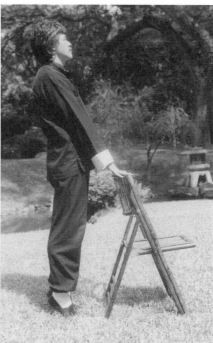

6

Crane Walking in the Clouds (Crane Form)— Standing with Chair Support Position

Step 1: STANDING WITH CHAIR SUPPORT: Lightly holding the back of a chair for support, lift your right heel. Press the ball of the foot into the ground and gently bending the right knee to keep your hips level. (Inhale.)

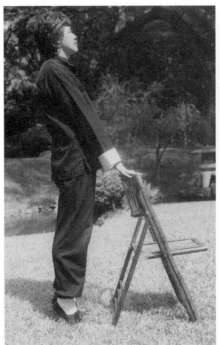 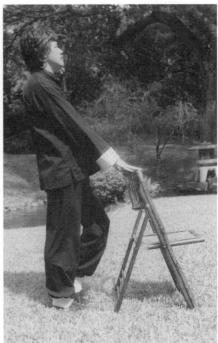

6

Crane Walking in the Clouds (Crane Form)—
Standing with Chair Support Position

Step 2: STANDING WITH CHAIR SUPPORT: Elevate both heels, balancing on the balls of both feet. Bring the right heel to the ground, leaving the left heel raised. Bend your left knee slightly to keep hips level. (Exhale.)

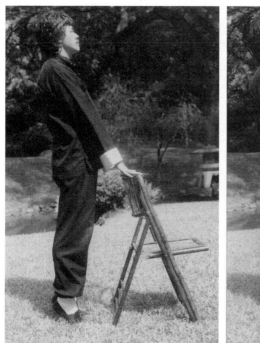
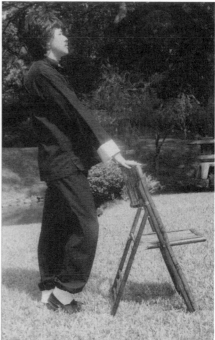

6

Crane Walking in the Clouds (Crane Form)— Standing with Chair Support Position

Step 3: STANDING WITH CHAIR SUPPORT: Elevate both heels again, balancing on the balls of both feet. Bring the left heel to the ground, leaving the right heel raised. Bend your right knee slightly to keep hips level. (Inhale.)

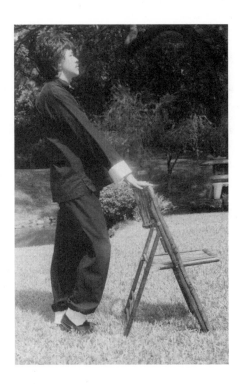

6

Crane Walking in the Clouds (Crane Form)—
Standing with Chair Support Position

Step 4: ENDING POSITION: You are now back at the starting position.

Repeat the exercise (Steps 1 through 3) 11 times, alternating the rise and fall of the right and left heels. Do vertical breathing throughout, remembering to begin the exercise at starting position with an inhale. Keep all movements slow and controlled.

Exercise 7

Rounding the Heaven and Earth Energy (Crane Form)

Rounding the Heaven and Earth Energy exercise creates a big circle using a single arm, then both arms. It can be done in a standing or seated position. While moving in clockwise and counterclockwise rotations, it is important here to move within the range of motion dictated by the flexibility of your shoulder joint. Do not push yourself beyond what is comfortable.

As always, breathing is important. The cosmic breath (chi) rides the flow of oxygen taken in through your nose, and the positioning of your body (legs, feet, back, arms, hands) adjusts your organs and meridians to accommodate healing energy flow.

This exercise balances yin and yang chi through the circular motion of your arms. The movements place your body in a number of beneficial feng shui postures, allowing healing energy into the system. Let yin chi lift your arm to the overhead position, and yang chi gently bring it down again.

Rounding Heaven and Earth Energy works to combat the ravages of osteoporosis, osteosclerosis, arthritis, and rheumatism, while strengthening the lungs and endocrine system. It also has been useful in the prevention and treatment of heart disease and breast cancer, along with relief from shoulder pain and stiffness.

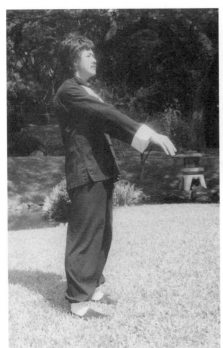
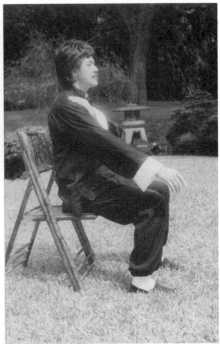

7-A

Rounding the Heaven and Earth Energy (Crane Form)

Step 1: STARTING POSITION: Stand or sit with feet shoulder-width distance apart, toes turned inward slightly. Place left hand on right shoulder. Extend the right arm downward to hip level. (Inhale and exhale.)

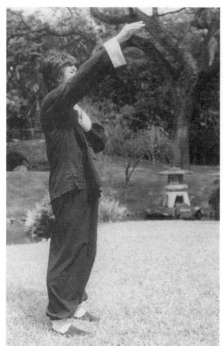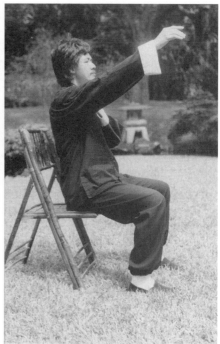

7-A

Rounding the Heaven and Earth Energy (Crane Form)

Step 2: Slowly circle your right arm clockwise, raising it to eye level, palm down. (Inhale until arm reaches your ear.)

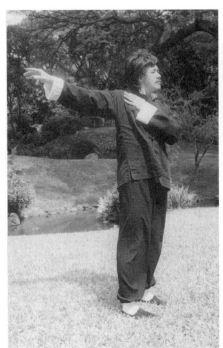 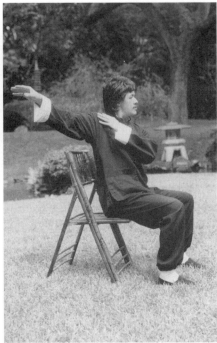

7-A

Rounding the Heaven and Earth Energy (Crane Form)

Step 3: Continue rotating your right arm overhead and toward the back, making the circle as large as possible. Bring your right arm down and back to the starting position, completing the circle. (Exhale until your arm returns to the starting position.)

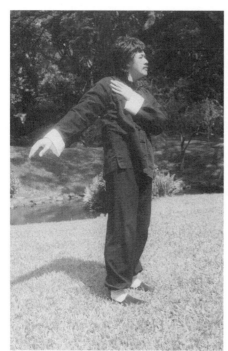 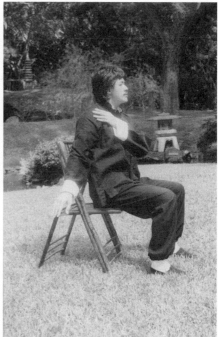

7-A

Rounding the Heaven and Earth Energy (Crane Form)

Step 4: Now work the same arm in a counter-clockwise direction, lifting to the back, overhead, and returning to the starting position again. Complete this movement 11 times, in both clockwise and counter-clockwise rotations. Change arms and repeat.

Do vertical breathing throughout, remembering to begin the exercise at starting position with an inhalation. Keep all movements slow and controlled.

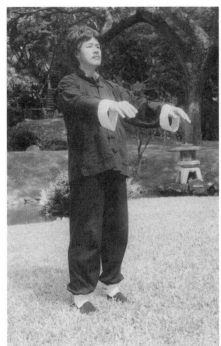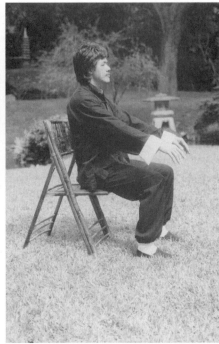

7-B

Rounding the Heaven and Earth Energy (Crane Form)

Step 1: STARTING POSITION: Stand or sit with feet shoulder-width distance apart, toes turned inward slightly. Extend both arms downward to hip level. (Inhale.)

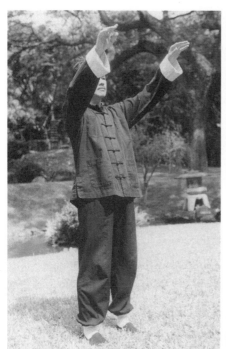
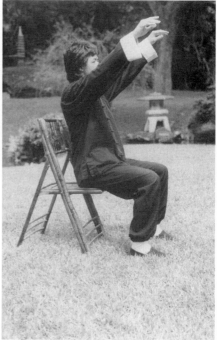

7-B

Rounding the Heaven and Earth Energy (Crane Form)

Step 2: Slowly circle your arms clockwise, raising them with palms down. (Inhale until arms reach your ears.)

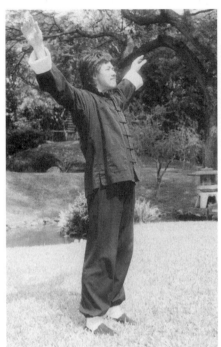 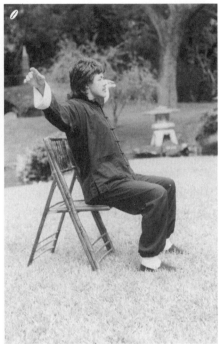

7-B

Rounding the Heaven and Earth Energy (Crane Form)

Step 3: Continue rotating your arms overhead and toward the back, making the circles as large as possible. (Exhale until your arms return to the starting position.)

Bring your arms down and back to the starting position, completing the circle. (Exhale.)

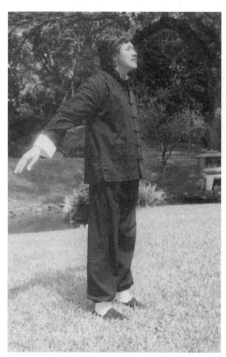 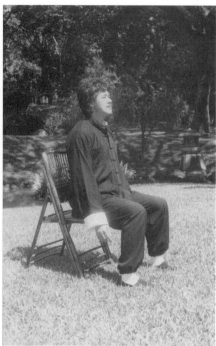

7-B

Rounding the Heaven and Earth Energy (Crane Form)

Step 4: Now work in a counter-clockwise direction, lifting to the back, overhead, and returning to the starting position again.

Complete this movement 11 times, in both clockwise and counter-clockwise rotations.

Do vertical breathing throughout, remembering to begin the exercise at starting position with an inhale. Keep all movements slow and controlled.

Exercise 8

Turning Over the Earth and Supporting the Sky with Both Arms

It isn't a very big job to roll the Earth and support the sky. The trick is in visualization. While doing this exercise imagine that you have the strength of Atlas, and that through the circular movements, you are rolling the earth and pushing against the sky, allowing chi to course through your body and out your palms.

Feel the heat of your blood running, flushing out the meridians, clearing the blocks that have collected through the years. There is invisible strength created by thought and images of the mind. And the name of this exercise tells you the types of feats you can accomplish with the help of this potent force.

Remember to concentrate on correct breathing, for breath is the means vital chi enters the body. The feng shui of this exercise affects physical balance, circulation, and fluidity of motion.

Turning Over the Earth and Supporting the Sky works to balance the inner ear, glucose/insulin exchange, and oxygen exchange in the lungs. In doing this the body adjusts to combat the effects of equilibrium loss, diabetes, and respiratory disease. The circulatory system, our body's nutrient lifeline, clears, and the painful stiffness of arthritis lessens.

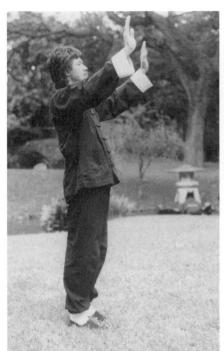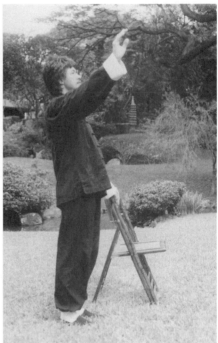

8

Turning Over the Earth and Supporting the Sky with Both Arms

Step 1: STARTING POSITION: Stand erect, lifting arms above your head. With or without the support of a chair, bend your knees, trying to keep your heels securely planted on the ground. Feet should be shoulder-width distance apart, toes turned inward slightly. The goal here is to get your thighs parallel to the ground.

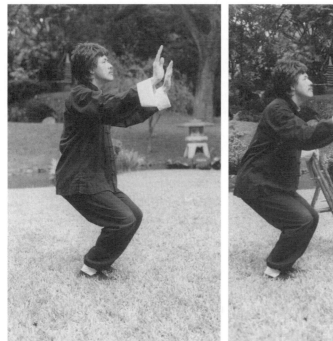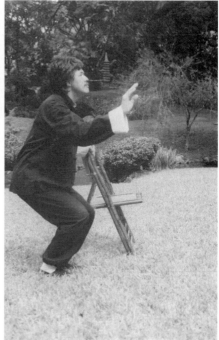

8

Turning Over the Earth and Supporting the Sky with Both Arms

Step 2: Bring both hands down near the ground, palms in the yin or down-facing position. Continue lowering your body and arms toward the earth. Imagine you are pushing and rolling a huge ball. (Inhale as you move down.)

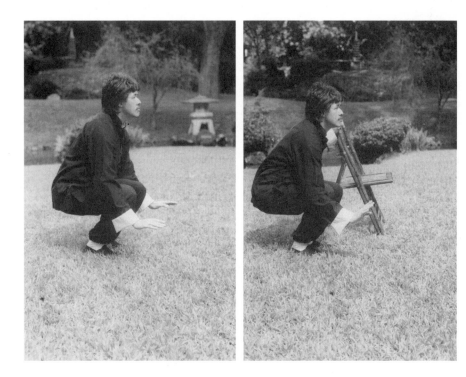

8

Turning Over the Earth and Supporting the Sky with Both Arms

Step 3: Keep your body erect, looking forward as you descend. Continue to inhale until you come to a full squat position with hands almost touching the ground. Move the air in a circular motion, both inside and outside of your body.

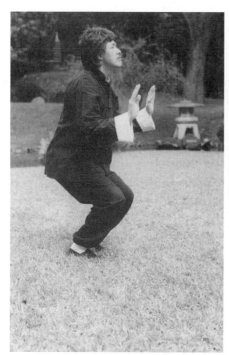 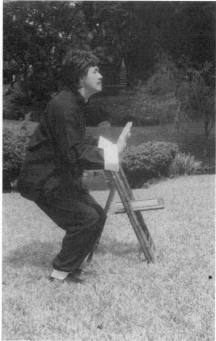

8

Turning Over the Earth and Supporting the Sky with Both Arms

Step 4: Continue the circular motion of the arms as you raise your body to an erect position. (Exhale while moving up.)

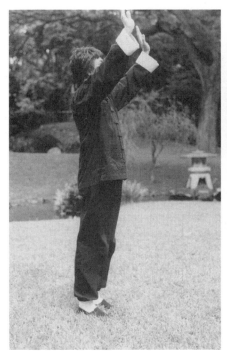
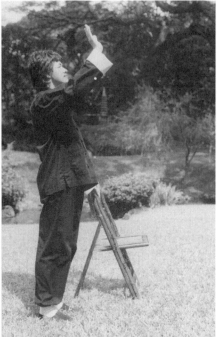

8

Turning Over the Earth and Supporting the Sky with Both Arms

Step 5: Raise your arms overhead, as if pushing up the sky.

Repeat the exercise sequence at least 11 times.

Exercise 9

Balancing the Earth (Neck Movement)

For most of us, life is a balancing act. Our minds are constantly reconciling our memories, justifying our daily experiences, and creating and recreating our dreams for the future. Through this process we find an equilibrium where our perception of the world, our personal planet Earth, can happily coexist with the rest of society.

The name of this exercise, Balancing the Earth, is a metaphor for our inner world of thoughts. Stress, one of modern man's most widespread afflictions, is created in the mind, causing meridian blocks that develop into headaches, a compromised immune system, and if left unchecked, serious disease.

Through a series of head rotations and concentrated deep breathing techniques, vital chi is allowed to flow through the blocked meridians. Once relaxed, the body is able to loosen and heal.

The movements can be done in a standing or seated position. Remember to keep your upper body still at all times during the movements, and to keep your feet firmly planted in the Earth.

Balancing the Earth relieves chronic migraine headaches, several types of ailments that cause stroke, the effects of Alzheimer's disease, arthritis, Parkinson's disease, and back and neck stiffness. It is also useful to relieve the nagging symptoms of the flu, and the unpleasant pain of a headache.

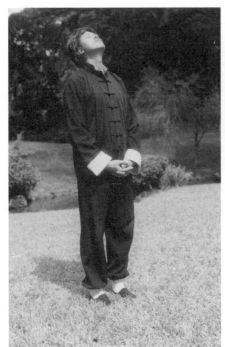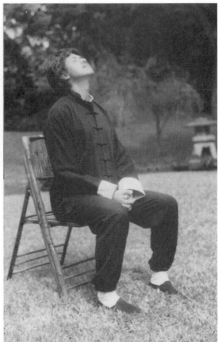

9-A

Balancing the Earth (Neck Movement)

Step 1: STARTING POSITION: Perform in a standing or seated position, feet shoulder-width distance apart, toes turned inward slightly. Clasp hands together, interlocking fingers, and rest in the dan tien area. Lift head up, toward sky, jaw raised, eyes closed. (Inhale.)

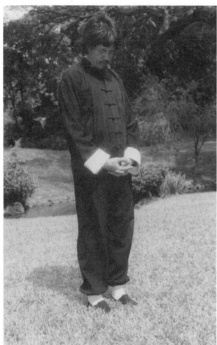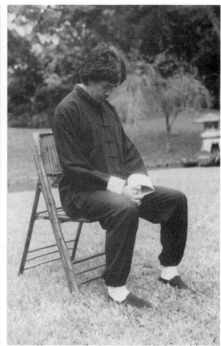

9-A

Balancing the Earth (Neck Movement)

Step 2: Lower head to look at the ground, jaw tucked into your chest. (Exhale.)

Repeat steps 1 and 2 at least 11 times.

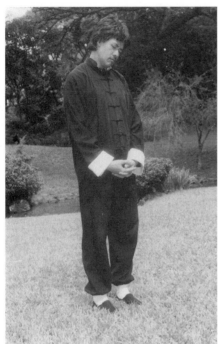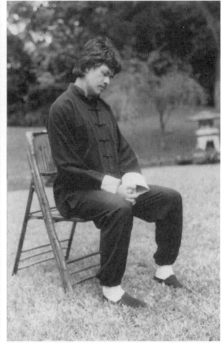

9-B

Balancing the Earth (Neck Movement)

Step 1: STARTING POSITION: Tilt your head to the left at a 45°
angle, and try to touch your chin to your collarbone. (Inhale.)

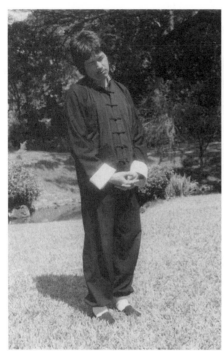 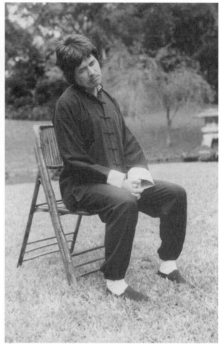

9-B

Balancing the Earth (Neck Movement)

Step 2: Straighten your head, then tilt it to the right at a 45° angle, touching your chin to the right side of your collarbone. (Exhale.)

Do steps 1 and 2 at least 11 times.

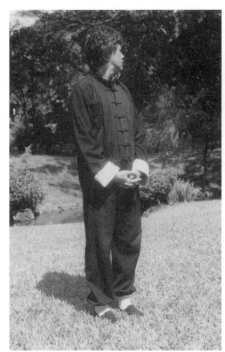
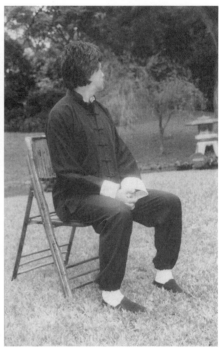

9-C

Balancing the Earth (Neck Movement)

Step 1: STARTING POSITION: Turn your head to look over your left shoulder. (Inhale.)

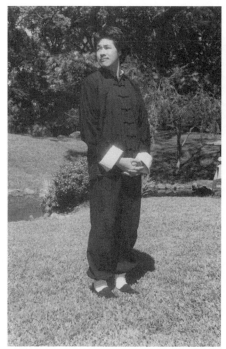 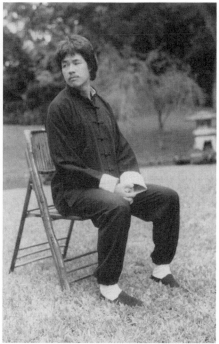

9-C

Balancing the Earth (Neck Movement)

Step 2: Now turn your head to look over your right shoulder. (Exhale.)

Do steps 1 and 2 at least 11 times.

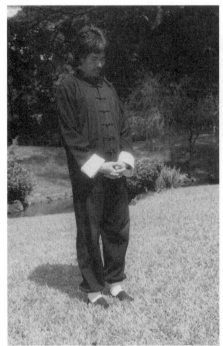 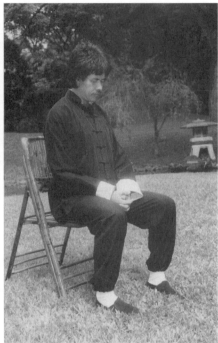

9-D

Balancing the Earth (Neck Movement)

Step 1: STARTING POSITION: Look down, focus on your dan tien breathing. Remain in this position for a while. (Inhale and exhale.)

Do step 1 at least 3 times before continuing to steps 2 through 4.

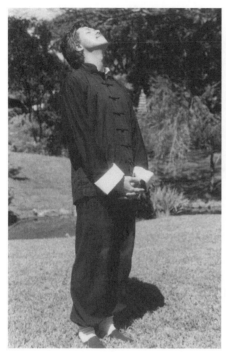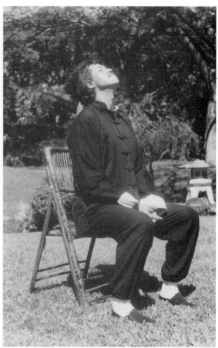

9-D

Balancing the Earth (Neck Movement)

Step 2: Gently turn your head up, facing the sky at a 45° angle.

Be sure to keep the movements slow and controlled, while gently moving the head in broad circles. Remember to inhale when moving to or from the left side of the body, and exhale when moving to or from the right.

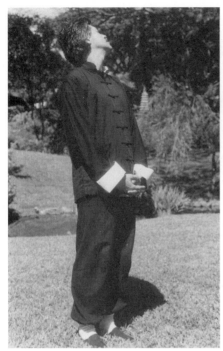 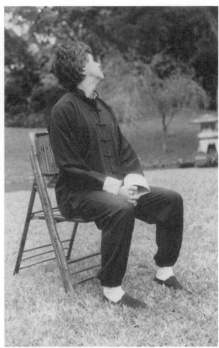

9-D

Balancing the Earth (Neck Movement)

Step 3: Then, slowly turn your head left. (Inhale.)

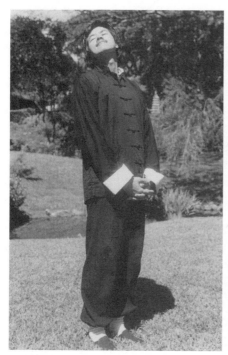 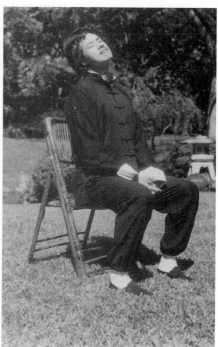

9-D

Balancing the Earth (Neck Movement)

Step 4: Slowly, turn your head to the right. (Exhale.)

Repeat steps 2 through 4 at least 11 times.

9-E
Balancing the Earth (Neck Movement)

Step 1: STARTING POSITION: Rotate your head and neck in a circular movement, 360° clockwise. Start inhaling as you move in the upward half of the circle. Exhale as you move through the downward half of circle.

9-E
Balancing the Earth (Neck Movement)

Step 2: Rotate your head and neck in a circular movement, 360° counter-clockwise. Inhale as you move through upward half of circle. Exhale as you move through the downward half of circle. (See photos on the following pages.)

Remember to do these movements at least 11 times in slow, controlled circles.

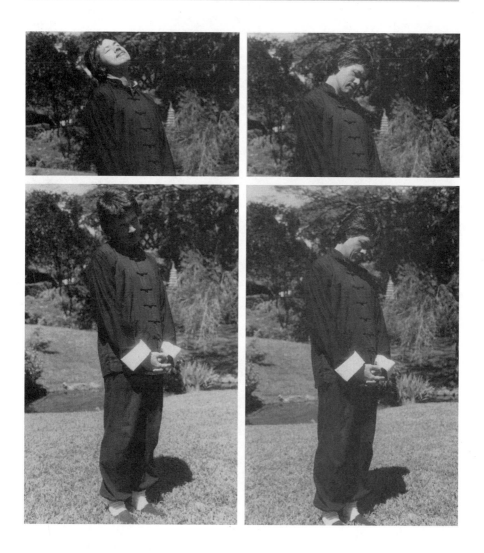

9-E

Balancing the Earth (Neck Movement)

Steps 1 and 2: Standing position.

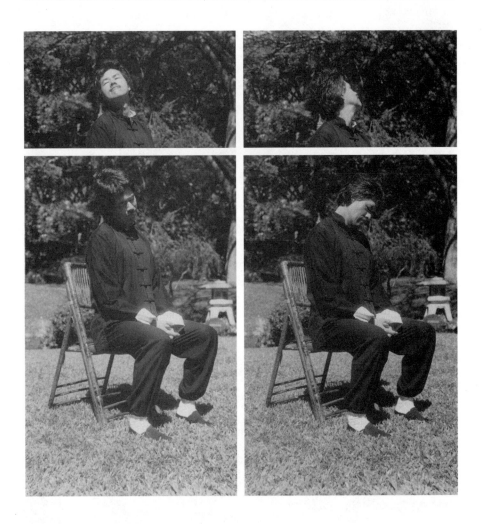

9-E

Balancing the Earth (Neck Movement)

Steps 1 and 2: Seated position.

Exercise 10

Tiger Eyes

T here are many factors that make working with chi both intriguing and baffling. First, it is difficult to measure chi even when using our most delicate scientific machinery. In China, scientists labor to either prove or disprove chi's existence. For me, the proof is in the individual healing I see taking place with my students.

One of the easiest exercises to do, although it is the strangest looking, is Tiger Eyes. You can do this anywhere, while working in an office, while relaxing with a favorite book, or even while sitting in a park. It is a rejuvenating exercise, designed to enliven the muscles of the face, and enhance eyesight.

I know that this can not be scientifically proven, but when one of my students turned 43, she was told she needed to wear glasses. It seems that the eyes get tired around the age of 40, and vision becomes blurred. I taught her to do the Tiger Eyes exercises, and instructed her to perform the movements as often as she could during the day. At first, she noticed that when she did the exercises, she could read perfectly. When she didn't do them, she couldn't see clearly. So, she practiced often. She has put her prescription glasses in a bottom desk drawer, and uses Tiger Eyes instead.

Remember, when doing this exercise, to keep the rest of your body relaxed. This helps your brain to focus. Visualize bringing chi through your body, and out through your eyes.

For centuries, the Chinese have used Tiger Eyes to improve both nearsightedness and farsightedness. One of the symptoms of diabetes is loss of eyesight. Tiger Eyes will help guard against this happening. The exercises also work to wake you up when you are drowsy. The Cat Washing the Face exercise actually helps prevent wrinkles.

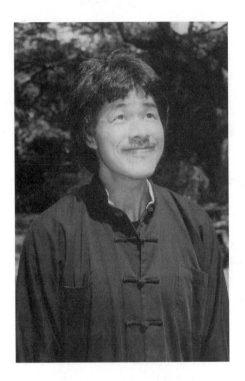

10-A
Tiger Eyes

Step 1: STARTING POSITION: This exercise can be done standing, sitting, or lying down. Open your eyes as wide as you can, and focus on a distant object. (Inhale.)

Visualize breathing through your eyes.

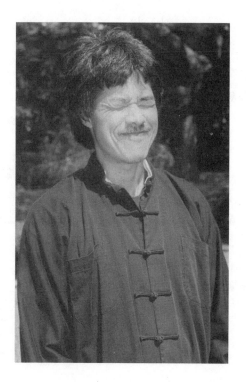

10-A

Tiger Eyes

Step 2: Close your eyes as tight as possible. (Exhale.)

Repeat exercise (Steps 1 and 2) at least 11 times, performing dan tien breathing throughout. Breathe through your eyes and nose.

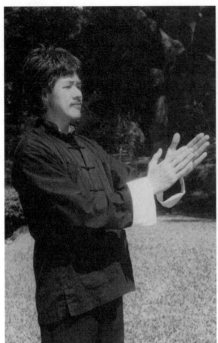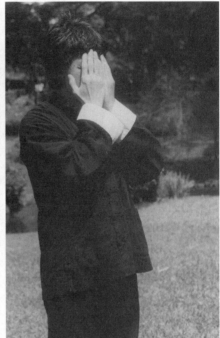

10-B
Cat Washing Face

Step 1: STARTING POSITION: Rub the palms of your hands together to generate chi energy. Place your hands on your upper cheeks. Feel the heat. (Inhale.)

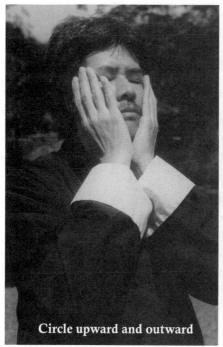

Circle upward and outward

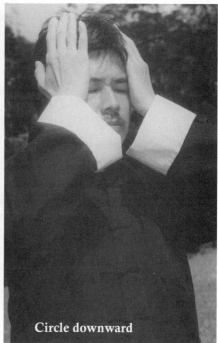

Circle downward

10-B
Cat Washing Face

Step 2: Circle your hands upward and outward around your eyes. Then downward, and back to the starting position. This is a natural face massage. Do not reverse the movement. Moving upward and outward helps prevent wrinkles. If you reverse the motion, it will move the chi against its natural flow, and will make more wrinkles. Repeat 11 times.

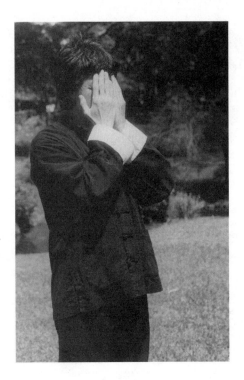

10-C
Cat Washing Face (Palms Cover Up the Eyes)

Step 1: STARTING POSITION: Do this exercise standing, sitting, or lying down.

Lightly cover eyes with the palms of your hands. Open your eyes wide, and inhale. Tightly close your eyes and exhale, receiving the energy. Repeat 11 times.

Perform dan tien breathing throughout.

Exercise 11

Eagle Looking for Food
(Mouth and Jaw Exercise)

I've noticed that in the West many people, both men and women, go to doctors for facelifts. It is an interesting thing to watch. In China, we use this specific chi exercise to tighten and tone sagging chin, neck, and jaw muscles to create a youthful countenance. Of course, exercises alone do not make a person look young. Diet, lots of water, sleep, and most importantly a youthful outlook generate the irresistible glow of youth.

This exercise is difficult to do, and if done incorrectly can be dangerous to your knees and back. Muscle strength and control is very important. Work at your own level. When bending, lean as far back as you can without experiencing pain. If it is too difficult, sit on a chair. It will support you where your muscles can not.

Remember to breathe in and out through your nose.

Eagle Looking for Food will relieve your back pain, strengthen your gums, and help to regulate your thyroid and saliva glands. It is a non-surgical way to get rid of that double chin, while firming up your profile, and helping to prevent wrinkles.

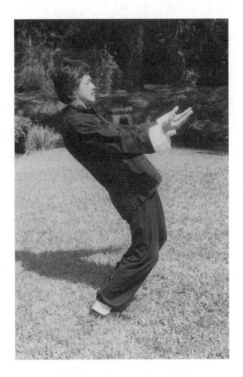

11
Eagle Looking for Food (Mouth and Jaw Exercise)

Step 1: STANDING POSITION: Plant your feet firmly on the ground, feet shoulder-width distance apart, toes turned slightly inward. Bend your knees and lean back to form curved bow. With palms in yang position, facing up, hold an imaginary chi ball in each hand. (Inhale.)

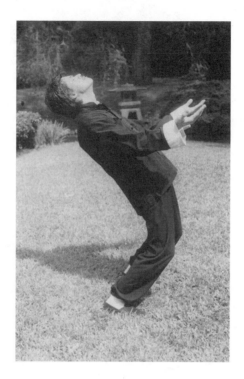

11

Eagle Looking for Food (Mouth and Jaw Exercise)

Step 2: STANDING POSITION: Tilt your head back as far as your muscles and balance will allow. (Exhale.)

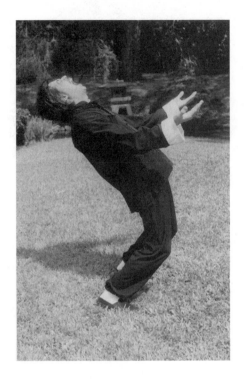

11

Eagle Looking for Food (Mouth and Jaw Exercise)

Step 3: STANDING POSITION: Open your mouth as wide as you can. (Inhale.)

Remember to breathe in through your nose.

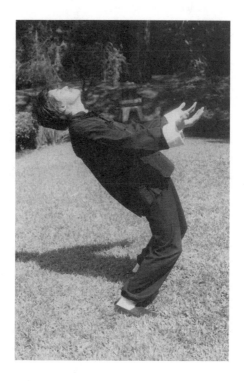

11

Eagle Looking for Food (Mouth and Jaw Exercise)

Step 4: STANDING POSITION: Close your mouth. (Exhale.)

Hold this position, opening and closing your mouth at least 11 times, or for as long as you can sustain the position. On the 11th time, and before straightening up, inhale once through your nose, and breathe out through both mouth and nose as if giving a loud yell.

Repeat this exercise (Steps 1 through 4) at least 11 times.

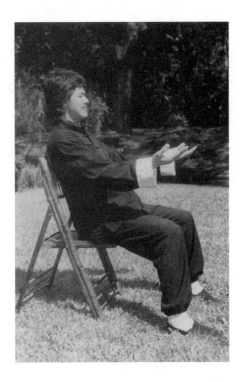

11

Eagle Looking for Food (Mouth and Jaw Exercise)

Step 1: SEATED POSITION: Position yourself at the edge of a chair. Plant your feet firmly on the ground, feet shoulder-width distance apart, toes turned slightly inward. Lean against the back of the chair, extending arms out in front of you. With palm in the yang position, facing up, hold an imaginary chi ball in each hand. (Inhale.)

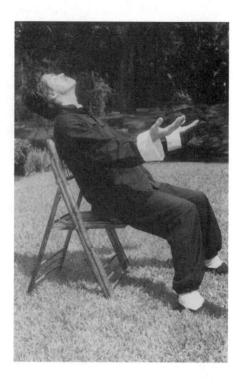

11

Eagle Looking for Food (Mouth and Jaw Exercise)

Step 2: SEATED POSITION: Tilt your head back as far as your muscles and balance will allow. (Exhale.)

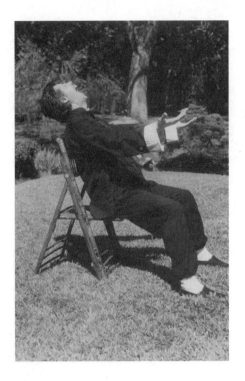

11

Eagle Looking for Food (Mouth and Jaw Exercise)

Step 3: SEATED POSITION: Open your mouth as wide as you can. Remember to breathe in through your nose. (Inhale.)

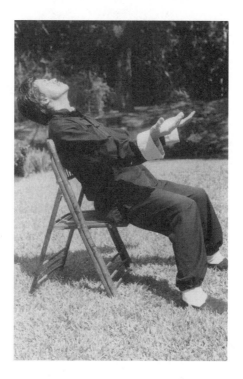

11

Eagle Looking for Food (Mouth and Jaw Exercise)

Step 4: SEATED POSITION: Close your mouth. (Exhale.)

Hold this position, opening and closing your mouth at least 11 times, or for as long as you can. On the 11th time, and before straightening up, inhale once through your nose, and breathe out through both mouth and nose as if giving a loud yell.

Repeat this exercise (Steps 1 through 4) at least 11 times.

Exercise 12

Cross Hands in Front of Face

This exercise demands flexibility of the hamstrings (the muscles located on the back of each thigh) and abdominals (stomach muscles). If you feel any discomfort during any part of the movement, feel free to modify how far you lean forward or back. Listen to your body. As you continue to practice, your muscles will get stronger, and you will be able to perform the exercises more freely.

Cross Hands in Front of Face is designed to improve the flexibility and strength of your back and abdominals, while opening the meridian channels that nourish the torso area. Bringing the hands toward the face initiates a beneficial feng shui alignment to help regulate the endocrine system. Because this exercise builds strength and stretches the low back and abdominal areas, it helps to relieve lower back pain and stiffness, and can even alleviate menstrual cramps.

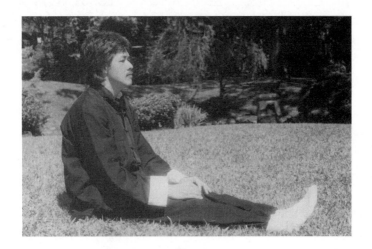

12

Cross Hands in Front of Face

Step 1: STARTING POSITION: Sit on the ground or floor, legs straight out in front of you. Place your hands on your knees. (Inhale and exhale.)

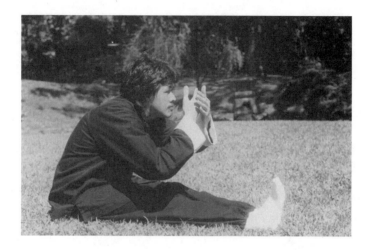

12

Cross Hands in Front of Face

Step 2: Lean forward from the hip, crossing both hands in front of your face. (Inhale and hold your breath.)

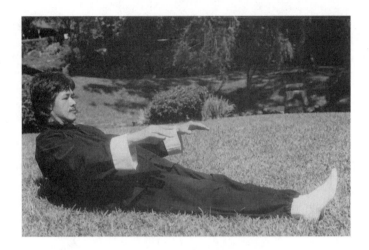

12

Cross Hands in Front of Face

Step 3: Lean back as far as your muscles will support, extending your hands forward, palms down. Try to keep your back as straight as possible. (Exhale.)

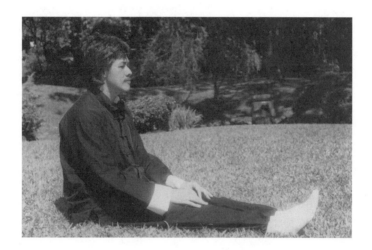

12

Cross Hands in Front of Face

Step 4: Return to upright seated position, hands resting comfortably on your knees. (Inhale.)

Repeat this series of movements at least 11 times, performing dan tien breathing throughout.

Exercise 13

Crane Catching the Fish

The visualization associated with this exercise is that of a crane, the symbol of longevity, swooping down to catch a fish for nourishment. This is also what you are doing, swooping down, gathering chi, and stimulating your internal organs, giving them nourishment.

At the apex of the movement of lifting your arms above your head, you are instructed to inhale. Visualize your ribcage stretching, elongating your torso, and providing essential breathing room for your internal organs. This movement causes air to be taken deep into the dan tien, and makes it possible to exhale twice (once in step 3 and once again in step 4) without needing another breath in between.

With the swooping movement, there is a tendency to let momentum carry the motion, instead of using muscle control. Be gentle with your body, and do not push yourself beyond your personal point of comfort. As you continue to practice these movements, your body will learn, and the exercises will become easier.

While doing the double exhalation, chi enters the body and cleanses the system. The overhead reach elongates the torso to allow your internal organs to stretch. It is kind of like lifting a rug to clean under and around it.

Crane Catching the Fish helps relieve lower back pain and stiffness, and calms menstrual cramps. The swooping movement of the torso assists in digestion and increases respiratory and endocrine system function. This exercise has also been used (with much success) to lessen the incidence of asthma, help people quit smoking, and open sinus passages.

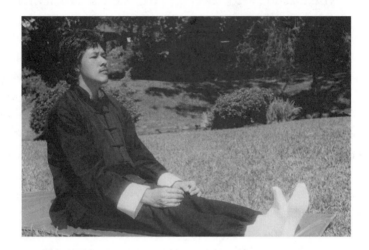

13

Crane Catching the Fish

Step 1: STARTING POSITION: Sit on the ground or floor, legs extended straight out in front of you, feet flexed. Lightly place your hands on your knees. (Inhale and exhale.)

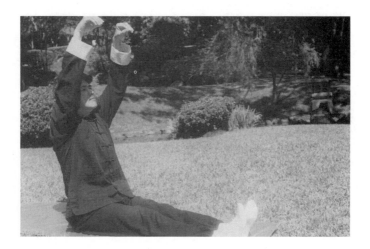

13

Crane Catching the Fish

Step 2: Keeping back straight, raise both arms overhead, closing fingers to make the beak of a crane. (Inhale.)

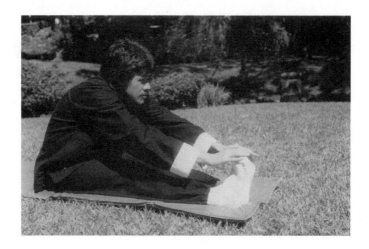

13

Crane Catching the Fish

Step 3: Lean forward, bending at the hip and gently curving the upper back, while pushing both hands toward your toes. (Exhale.)

If you can't touch your toes, push your hands as close to them as possible without causing pain. As you practice, you will become more flexible.

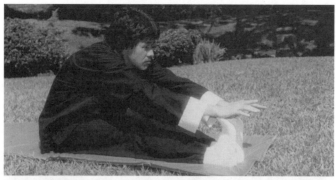

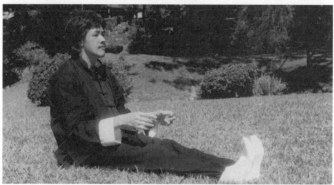

13

Crane Catching the Fish

Step 4: Pull back slightly, holding your breath. Lean forward again, bending even deeper through the hip, while pushing both hands past your toes. (Exhale.)

There is a double exhale, once in step 3, letting out some of your air, and once again in step 4. On this second push, the goal is to push both hands farther forward, touching the tips of your toes with your wrists.

Repeat this series at least 11 times, performing dan tien breathing throughout.

Exercise 14

Secret Fountain of Youth
(Timeless Mind and Ageless Body)

While doing this exercise, visualize a crane curling its feet in the mud for balance. Done in a seated position, the Secret Fountain of Youth clears the meridians and channels of the extremities of the arms and legs.

All hand and feet motions are done simultaneously—when curling your toes, you are making fists with your hands; when spreading your fingers, you are spreading your toes. Remember the fluid movements of the crane, beautifully balanced both in flight and on the ground.

As chi is taken into the body through the nose, sent down to the dan tien, then up through the meridians and channels to the hands and feet, it nourishes all of the organs and glands along the way. This exercise improves digestion, respiratory function, and nervous system conduction, while enhancing the endocrine and immune systems. The rotation of the hands and feet also relieves inflamed and stiff hand and foot joints caused by arthritis. (Refer to hand and foot illustrations on pages 108 and 110.)

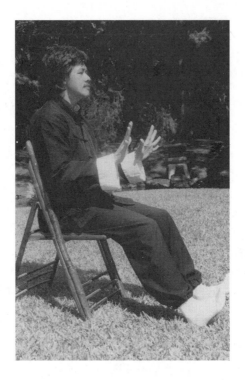

14-A

Secret Fountain of Youth (Timeless Mind and Ageless Body)

Step 1: STARTING POSITION: Sit on a chair with back straight. Flex both feet, pointing toes upward. Bend elbows at 90° angles, wrists flexed, fingers spread. (Inhale.)

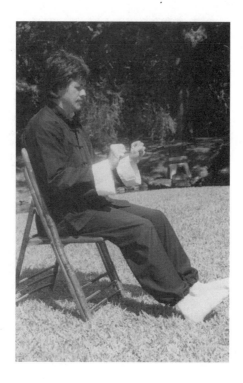

14-A

Secret Fountain of Youth (Timeless Mind and Ageless Body)

Step 2: Crunch toes downward, keeping feet flexed. Make tight fists with your hands, holding elbows stationary. (Exhale.)

Repeat steps 1 and 2 at least 11 times.

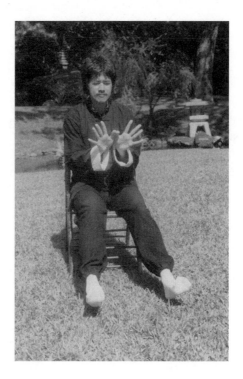

14-B

Secret Fountain of Youth (Timeless Mind and Ageless Body)

Step 1: STARTING POSITION: Bringing thumbs together, spread fingers as wide as possible. With feet still flexed, point toes upward again. (Inhale.)

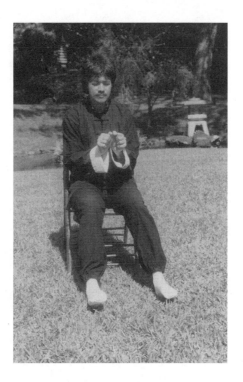

14-B

Secret Fountain of Youth (Timeless Mind and Ageless Body)

Step 2: Keeping thumbs together, make fists with both hands, and crunch toes again. (Exhale.)

Repeat steps 1 and 2 at least 11 times.

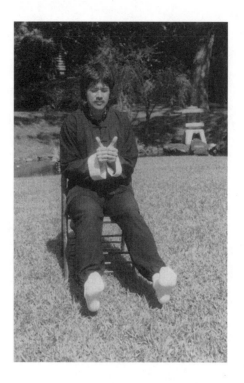

14-C

Secret Fountain of Youth (Timeless Mind and Ageless Body)

Step 1: STARTING POSITION: Press toes and thumbs up, keeping fingers in fist. (Inhale.)

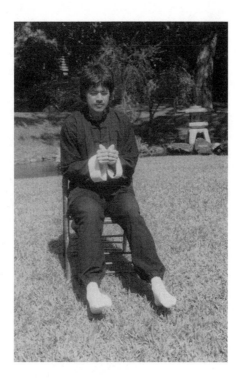

14-C

Secret Fountain of Youth (Timeless Mind and Ageless Body)

Step 2: Crunch toes, and press thumbs down. (Exhale.)

Repeat steps 1 and 2 at least 11 times.

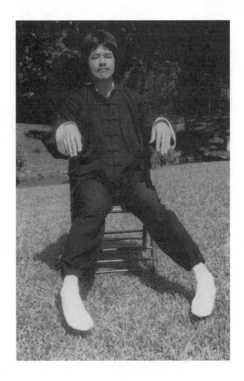

14-D

Secret Fountain of Youth (Timeless Mind and Ageless Body)

Step 1: STARTING POSITION: Open your hands, pointing fingers downward. Extend feet, toes pointed slightly inward. (Inhale.)

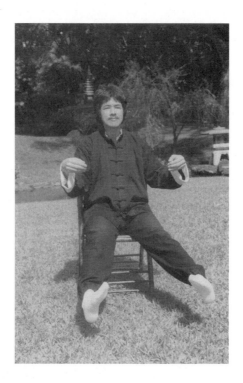

14-D

Secret Fountain of Youth (Timeless Mind and Ageless Body)

Step 2: Circle hands and feet clockwise, moving inward and up at the beginning of each rotation. When your toes and hands are pointing up, inhale. When they are pointing down, exhale.

Repeat steps 1 and 2 at least 11 times. Repeat movements counterclockwise, at least 11 times.

Exercise 15

Bending Knees on Floor (Crane Form)

Bending Knees on Floor is another crane form exercise. When developing the concepts and movements that eventually became known as t'ai chi and chi kung, Cheung San Fung watched the graceful motions and postures of animals in his environment that possessed the gift of longevity. One of the important things he discovered was that if the cosmic energy of chi was combined with movements imitating these animals, the meridians in the body would open. In addition to this, he realized that practicing fluid movements increased flexibility, which allowed more fluidity of motion. When the body moved with more grace, the mind was more relaxed. This, then, was both internally and externally beneficial.

The spine, the most valuable support structure in our bodies, is also the most abused. Sitting in static postures for long periods of time (in front of a computer for hours), or with improper body alignment, compromises the spine, which then stiffens. Once this happens, our entire system feels the pain—we walk bent over, stand crooked, sit hunched, and eventually, if the problems are not corrected, we block our meridians and become ill.

This exercise is a way to increase flexibility in the lower back, torso, and hips, the foundation blocks of our physical structure.

The Bending Knees on Floor exercise works to improve lower back strength and flexibility, while strengthening the bones, and slimming the torso. Through controlled twisting of the waist, pain and stiffness are relieved.

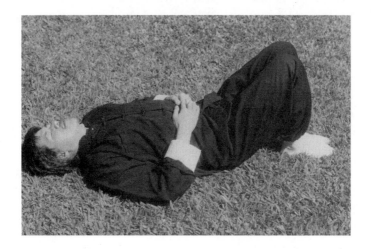

15

Bending Knees on Floor (Crane Form)

Step 1: STARTING POSITION: Lie on floor, feet together, knees bent, hands on your abdomen. Relax your shoulders and back. (Inhale and exhale.)

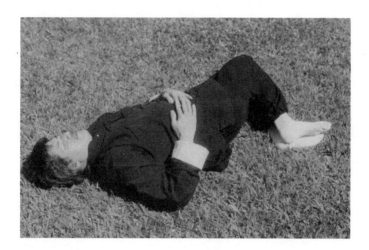

15

Bending Knees on Floor (Crane Form)

Step 2: Keeping the upper body relaxed, feet together, shoulders square and flat against the ground, twist your torso to allow your knees to fall to the left. (Inhale.)

The goal of this movement is to rest your knees on the ground, but if that is not possible at this time, twist as far as possible without discomfort or pain. Shoulders must remain on the floor.

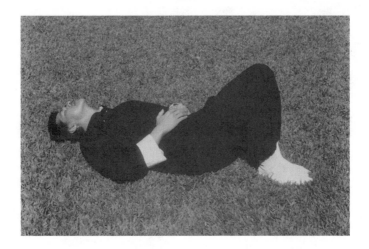

15

Bending Knees on Floor (Crane Form)

Step 3: Raise knees to upright position. (Exhale.)

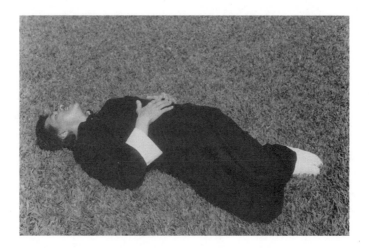

15

Bending Knees on Floor (Crane Form)

Step 4: Again, keeping the upper body relaxed, feet together, shoulders square and flat against the ground, twist your torso to allow your knees to fall to the right. (Inhale.)

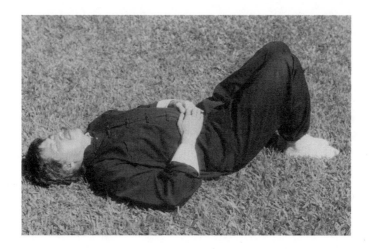

15

Bending Knees on Floor (Crane Form)

Step 5: Return to starting position and begin the movement over again. (Exhale.)

Repeat Steps 1 to 5 at least 11 times.

Perform dan tien breathing throughout.

Exercise 16

The Inner Treasure of Meditation (Sitting Meditation)

The next chapter, entitled **Moving the Chi Within,** provides four meditations designed to calm, enliven, or heal. Choose one of these to use as your 16th chi exercise.

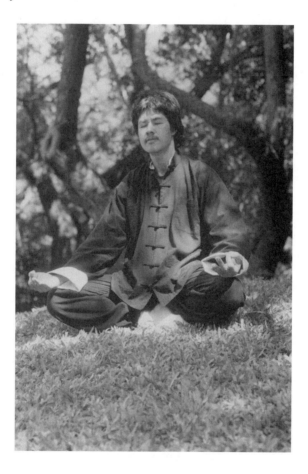

Moving the Chi Within

In teaching meditation, I emphasize the visualization of light, for that is what chi is, the light of life, the shining breath.

Many who have practiced yoga and New Age meditation will be familiar with some of the techniques revealed in this chapter. The difference is visualization, which enhances energy movement through the meridians and channels of the body. Coupled with the movements of chi kung, it is possible to physically position the body into postures that enhance the healing effects of chi.

During the calm of meditation the mind focuses on the chi we take in with each breath, gently blends it with the jung chi generated by our bodies, then moves it up the spine, through the meridians, and into the channels and extremities. All of this is done with concentration on correct breathing technique (dan tien breathing) and simple mind control.

Chi is the foundation that builds a strong and powerful mind (internal self) and body (external self). Although dynamic by nature, the movement of chi can be controlled. Sitting meditation is an excellent way to quiet the mind and focus chi energy.

With each inhalation, remember to collect the air in the lower abdomen (dan tien). Breathing deeply into the diaphragm increases the amount of oxygen supply to the blood, and rejuvenates the system to produce a sense of well-being. Visualize the chi as a radiant ball of silvery light. As you progress in the meditation steps, you will learn to move this ball, illuminating the meridians along the way until your entire body fills with fluorescent chi energy. All of this helps to awaken cerebral powers, and enliven the tired psyche.

My students sometimes find it difficult to relax enough to feel the effects of the tranquil minutes of meditation. In these cases I suggest playing soft, mellow music. The body relaxes with slow rhythms. The vibrations create an atmosphere of peace for the mind to release the stresses of the day. In this quiet state, tension loosens, muscles unwind, circulation improves, and blood pressure drops.

One day, a 35-year-old man showed up at one of our morning exercise sessions. He arrived at the park with his friend, a regular student, but he wouldn't participate in the exercises. For most of the hour Stanley (not his real name) stood in the back of the class with his arms folded over his chest. He watched the other students work their way through a very simple chi kung routine.

I always pay attention to the dynamics of group work. It is difficult for the untrained eye to follow the movement of chi through a landscape in nature, but watching chi move through a crowd of people is very easy. When people start to relax, they subconsciously move away from stagnant or agitated chi, creating space between themselves and the source of the uncomfortable energy.

Once the class started, I noticed a broadening semicircle of space pushing through the students. At the center of the semicircle stood pent-up Stanley, leaning against a tree. His lips were pursed, eyes narrowed, jaw clenched. About half-way through the class, he started to pace, looking at his watch. His friend, a lovely young lady, continued with her exercises. She, like the rest of the students, had moved far enough away from him to allow the creation of her own environment of calm. She came to class often, and as was her custom, she stood next to an 81-year-old woman we nicknamed "Little Angel." Little Angel is a class favorite. She exudes a loving, nurturing energy that attracts everyone. She is like sweet nectar on a dew-drenched flower. Everyone loves her.

Stanley finally walked away, out of sight. He returned moments later, as we were preparing to complete the class with our standard meditation practice. I instructed the students to get their mats or blankets, and sit cross-legged on the ground. To my surprise, Stanley walked into the circle and plopped down.

"Very well," I said. "Let us begin the meditation." I walked to the tape recorder and switched on some soft music. "For those of you who are new with us today, place one hand on your chest, and one hand on your diaphragm. Close your eyes. Let your tongue naturally rest on the roof of your mouth, and breathe through your nose." I could feel the group relax right away. "Take the air from each breath, and push it down to fill your diaphragm. Let your belly swell, then exhale through your nose. The hand on your chest should remain still, while the hand on your diaphragm should slowly rise and fall as the abdomen fills and deflates." I watched a gentle calm settle over the class. "Continue this breathing."

I looked at Stanley. He was in the most interesting posture. He sat correctly, his hands where I told him to put them, and his diaphragm was expanding and contracting. But his shoulders were lifted almost to his ears, like he was fighting internal pain. I walked to the back of the class, then up behind Stanley. Inhaling to focus my chi, I put my hands three inches above his shoulders and began to draw his shoulders outwards and down. "Keep breathing," I said. It took a while, but soon Stanley's upper body slumped, and in moments he was listing, as his relaxed body drifted in a half-conscious sleep.

After class, Stanley and his friend waited to speak to me. "I feel like I've had a solid 8 hours of sleep," Stanley said. "It feels like a Sunday morning." He held out his hand. "Thank you."

I took his hand and gave a friendly shake. "You need to come back many times," I told him. "You can feel that way every day, all day."

"I just came here because she wanted me to," he said, pointing to his friend.

"Yes," I said. "Good. But you should come to class often."

"Maybe I'll show up near the end of the class just for the meditation," he said. "Then I don't have to wait around. My doctor says that I have to relax because of my rashes and ulcers. He said I should look into some kind of meditation, so I thought I'd try this."

"You come and do the chi kung exercises," I said. "The meditation will help you relax, but the chi is blocked in your body, and you have already created illnesses. You should do the chi kung exercises, too. It's like when you have a headache. You take aspirin to alleviate the pain right away, but there might be something else wrong, an illness that is really causing the headache, so you must go see a doctor. You are all the time feeling stress. You have been this way for a long time. OK. Now you do the meditation, and you feel better. It's like the aspirin. You need to come and do the chi kung to fix the rest of the illness. We will see you tomorrow."

Stanley came back the next day, and has attended every class for two years. His ulcers are gone, so are the rashes, and he meditates at least once a day.

There are four styles of meditation introduced in this chapter.

The **first** meditation is a seated version of dan tien breathing. Refer back to these techniques whenever necessary.

The **second** series of exercises—Awakening the Tiger—is designed to wake up the mind, drive away any drowsiness, and enliven the jung chi of the body. Doing this meditation in the morning prepares you for the day by gently invigorating your system, and sharpening your thought processes. It creates a focused vitality.

The **third** series—Quieting the Dragon—helps to calm the mind, and bring about a peaceful feeling. Our hectic schedules often deprive us of needed sleep, and often cause worry-racked insomnia. But a short period of quiet meditation before bedtime releases the anxiety, and produces the relaxing drift needed to rest. This style of meditation is also used in China to relieve stress-induced pain.

The **fourth** and final series—the Meditation for Longevity and Health—is for healing, and the visualization techniques will help you locate and concentrate on areas of your body that need special attention. When you do this type of meditation, and are sensitive to your body's subtle language, you'll find blocks that were created by emotional stress and old emotional wounds. These are important to clear, because these blocks in the meridians precipitate illness.

I've found that healing occurs in stages. With each cleared meridian blockage, another, deeper scar will be found in the same spot. Daily clearing and attention to these blocks will release trapped emotions, one at a time, until the illness is finally healed. These trapped emotions are the dark thoughts and attitudes, the suppressed worries and psychic pain that started the blocks in the first place. This meditation may bring up long forgotten feelings of hurt and anger. Allow yourself to remember them. Let the tears flow. They are your body's physical expression of release. They will wash away the clutter and refresh your spirit.

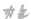

I've presented these meditations in steps. Each step will take some practice. Be patient with yourself. Any effort, even the ones you feel have failed, will greatly benefit your health and well-being.

Once you've learned to do the basic steps, move onto the next. This process may take weeks, even months. Don't worry. Your body will feel the effects right away. Any movement of chi through the system will create a blossoming of beneficial results.

These meditation techniques are very similar. They all include the visualization of light coupled with dan tien breathing. The differences are very subtle, but meaningful. You will feel the health benefits, no matter when you decide to meditate.

Location. Consult the previous chapter for advice about the feng shui of where to locate your meditation. Privacy is important for some students, and they prefer to be at home, alone in a room.

Seated Dan Tien Breathing Technique

a. Sit cross-legged on the floor in classic meditation posture: back straight, hands on your knees, palms up, with the tip of each thumb and pointing finger touching (this forms a circle to hold a small chi ball in each hand).

b. Close your eyes and mouth. Breathe through your nose.

c. Place your tongue against your palate, and focus on bringing air in through your nose.

d. Visualize the air going down into your diaphragm (two inches below the navel).

e. Place one hand on your chest; fingers spread. (This hand should not move as you breathe. If your chest is rising and falling, you are not breathing correctly.)

f. Place the other hand on your abdomen, thumb over belly-button and four fingers slightly spread over the lower abdomen.

g. Breathe in through the nose, expanding the diaphragm and bringing the air into the dan tien. (As you inhale, air should fill the lower abdominal cavity, creating a rounded, balloon-like bulge. This is called "filling the dan tien.")

h. Hold this posture for 2 seconds. If you feel lightheaded at any time, reduce the time held to 1 second.

i. Visualize the air in your abdomen as a collection of light; a glowing ball.

j. Exhale through the nose.

k. Repeat the breathing sequence, concentrating on correct technique, for a minimum of 6 minutes, and work up to 20 minutes each meditation session.

NOTE: This all happens very quickly with one breath. Don't try to have the visualization with the first breath you take using this technique. Concentrate on the breathing. It may take some practice. Be patient. Stay calm. This is a skill worth learning well.

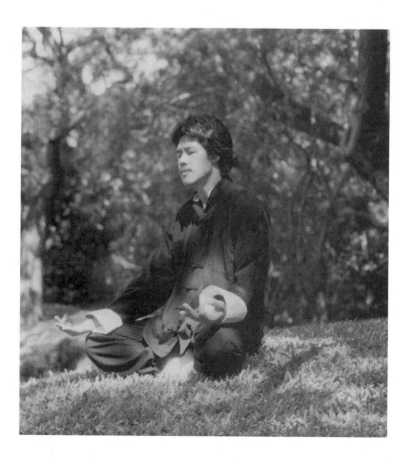

Awakening the Tiger (morning meditation)

This meditation can be done after you have completed your morning chi kung exercises, or as you rise from sleep.

Follow the dan tien breathing technique described above in steps a through j. **Continue this slow, deep breathing throughout the meditation.**

Visualize the glowing chi ball in your lower abdomen.

As you exhale, move the "ball" downward to your tailbone, then upward along your spine, into your skull, then out through your nose.

Repeat this at least 3 times and increase as you become more comfortable with this process. You will experience a strengthening energy force throughout your entire body as your jung chi is enlivened.

Release any thoughts as they come into your mind, and concentrate on moving the ball of light.

Feel the energy in your chest, down your arms and legs and bring the light into your fingers and toes.

Some people physically feel the chi warmth. Don't worry if you start to sweat. This is a favorable response.

Repeat this breathing and visualization for up to 20 minutes. It may take some practice before you feel completely comfortable, but it's worth the effort.

As you complete the meditation, take in one final dan tien breath, raise your arms above your head, palms facing upward, and collect the yang energy of the heavens.

You are ready to start your day.

Quieting the Dragon (evening meditation)

This meditation can be done after you have completed your evening chi kung exercises, or when your house is quiet, and you are preparing to go to bed.

It is best to do this meditation lying down. Place your hands beside your body, palms down. Once your body is totally relaxed, you won't want to get up.

Begin with the dan tien breathing described above in dan tien breathing technique, steps a through j. **Continue this slow, deep breathing throughout the meditation.**

Visualize the glowing chi ball in your lower abdomen.

As you exhale, move the "ball" downward to your tailbone, then upward along your spine, into your skull, then out through your nose.

Repeat this at least 3 times. Increase the number of breaths as you become more comfortable with this process.

Quiet the mind by releasing any thoughts that come into your head, and focus on moving the ball of light.

You will experience a slight tingling as the chi courses through your body and your jung chi balances with your breathing.

Continue the dan tien breathing.

Move the energy into your chest, then concentrate on pushing out all tension from your shoulders and arms, letting the chi wash like a bath of light through the upper half of your body.

Continue to pulse the chi light through the channels of your shoulders and arms until the area tingles and you feel a warm glow.

Now, begin to fix your concentration on the lower half of your body.

Move the energy from your chest, through the meridians in your torso, down your legs, all the way to your toes, pushing the tension out the through your feet.

Some people report a liquid warmth in their limbs, as if the muscles and bones become fluid and pliant.

Maintain the dan tien breathing throughout the meditation while guiding the chi energy deeper and deeper into your body, relaxing every organ, tendon, muscle, and joint.

Repeat this breathing and visualization for about 20 minutes. It may take some practice before you feel comfortable, but it's worth the effort.

As you complete your meditation time, take in one final dan tien breath. Feel the weight of your body sink into the mattress. Adjust your head on the pillow.

For a moment, focus on your down-turned palms. Collect the nurturing yin energy of Mother Earth, the balancing element to the yang activities of your work day.

Good Night.

Meditation for Longevity and Health (healing meditation)

We have talked at length about the effect that blocked meridians have on the health and well-being of internal organs. This meditation is designed to help you feel the areas where your meridians are blocked. It is important to be sensitive to any difficulty you have moving the light through your body, and to any aches or pains you encounter. If this happens, concentrate the chi light in that area until you feel a release, or the flow seems to begin again. You may find that the blocks will need repeated clearing. Patience and focus are essential. Remember that it has taken a long time to build these blocks, so it may take concentrated effort and perseverance to free them.

Sit, back erect, on a chair, or cross-legged on the floor. Place your hands, palms up, on your thighs, as close to your knees as is comfortable. Lightly touch the tip of each thumb and pointing finger together.

Begin with the dan tien breathing described above in dan tien breathing technique, steps a through j. **Continue this slow, deep breathing throughout the meditation.**

Visualize the glowing chi ball in your lower abdomen.

As you exhale, move the "ball" downward to your tailbone, then upward along your spine, into your skull, then out through your nose.

Breathe deeply into the dan tien, concentrating on the chi as it enters your body.

Quiet your mind by releasing any thoughts that come into your head, and focus on moving the ball of light.

You will experience a slight tingling as the chi courses through your body and your jung chi intensifies.

Continue the dan tien breathing.

Move the energy into your chest, focusing on the central core of your torso, then slowly maneuver the golden chi ball down the front of your body. Pay close attention to any blocks or spots where the chi passage seems to slow or stop.

When you find a block or obstruction, hold the chi light in that area. As you continue your dan tien breathing, intensify the light, filling the entire space with chi.

Some people have experienced slight pain when they concentrate the light in a meridian region. If this happens to you, stay with it. Continue the deep breathing until the irritation subsides. Old wounds need gentle patience.

Remember, it may take several meditation periods to release a serious blockage. Be patient with yourself, and know that this healing work has the power to reverse potentially serious problems.

Don't worry if, on the first try or second, you are unable to release the blocked energy. You will meditate tomorrow, and it will get easier the more you practice.

A cleared block feels like a gentle drop into deeper relaxation. When you feel this, continue to move the chi ball down the mid-line of your torso, stopping whenever needed to work on obstructions.

I have included a diagram of the meridians and channels to provide a visual "map" of chi flow. From the torso, take the ball of light down both legs, letting the energy radiate from your feet.

Fill your torso and legs with chi light, and continue the dan tien breathing.

Collect another ball of light in the lower abdomen and move it up your spine as before. This time, work the chi through your arms.

Visualize the light shooting out from the tips of your fingers and the center of your palms.

Your body should radiate with life force. Enjoy the warmth.

During this period, visualize a pulsing energy in the areas where blocks were found. Let the light work to clear any barriers.

You can do this meditation for as long as your schedule permits. It is not important that you experience all of the feelings and sensations described above. Our bodies speak to us in many different ways. Learn to listen, and communicate.

Take your time, be patient. Good health sometimes needs a little coaxing.

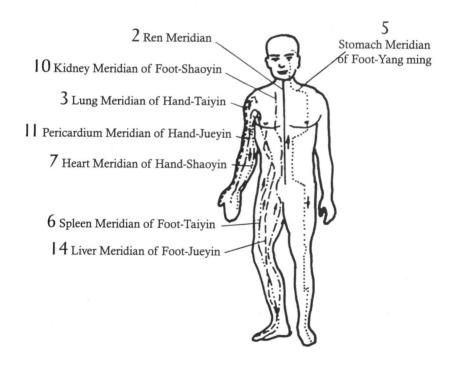

2 Ren Meridian

5
Stomach Meridian of Foot-Yang ming

10 Kidney Meridian of Foot-Shaoyin

3 Lung Meridian of Hand-Taiyin

11 Pericardium Meridian of Hand-Jueyin

7 Heart Meridian of Hand-Shaoyin

6 Spleen Meridian of Foot-Taiyin

14 Liver Meridian of Foot-Jueyin

Location of the Points of the Fourteen Meridians (Part 1)

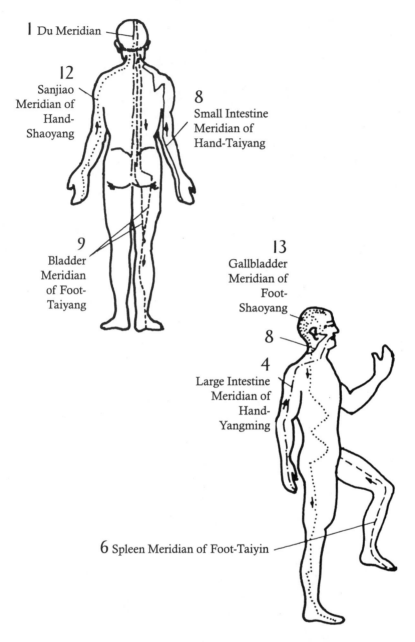

1 Du Meridian

12
Sanjiao
Meridian of
Hand-
Shaoyang

8
Small Intestine
Meridian of
Hand-Taiyang

9
Bladder
Meridian
of Foot-
Taiyang

13
Gallbladder
Meridian of
Foot-
Shaoyang

8

4
Large Intestine
Meridian of
Hand-
Yangming

6 Spleen Meridian of Foot-Taiyin

Location of the Points of the Fourteen Meridians (Parts 2 & 3)

The Green Diet of Chi

"Trouble and problems come out of our mouths. Sickness starts with what we put into our mouths."—Chinese proverb

The goal for anyone taking t'ai chi and chi kung is to develop a sound mind and body for a longer, happier, and healthier life. In order to achieve this goal, we work to create a balance of yin and yang chi both inside and outside our bodies. Earlier chapters have concentrated on the physical means of achieving this goal, manipulating the feng shui of our external world and the feng shui and chi movement within our bodies. Another very important element is balancing the chi taken into our systems through diet.

The *I Ching* (the secret book) talks about nutrition and how it complements and balances the healing arts of t'ai chi and chi kung. The *I Ching* promises that through this balance, one can learn the secrets of the fountain of youth, of longevity and health, and of feng shui, "the martial arts against illness."

Jung chi, generated within our bodies by our thoughts, emotions, and attitudes, is greatly affected by what we eat. There is an ancient Chinese saying, "Let food be your medicine. We are what we put into our mouths." Foods, according to the Chinese, are classified into three categories: the Yin (negative energy), Yang (positive energy), and Neutral. Yang foods are believed to be responsible for what the Chinese refer to as hot or inflammatory diseases like swollen glands, allergies, fevers, cancers (especially colon cancer, prostate cancer, and breast cancer), constipation, hemorrhoids, and the inflammation and infection of internal organs. Yin foods are calming to the mind, as well as the body. And Neutral foods act as an inert base that assists in balancing both yin and yang. Obviously, foods from the Neutral category are best for everyday consumption, and are the recommended choices. In all dietary considerations, remember to be moderate. As my father would often say, "Everything in moderation, including moderation itself."

We call this diet the "Green Diet" because it emphasizes the Earth-greens of the Yin and Neutral food categories, as opposed to the heavy Yang intake of most Western diets. Green is also the color of growth, or the spiraling up toward health.

In the Green Diet you should endeavor to eat more Yin and Neutral foods to balance out the powerful Yang foods. It is that simple.

Examples of foods in the various categories are shown in the following table:

YIN FOOD	YANG FOOD	NEUTRAL FOOD
bananas	alcohol	apples
barley	asparagus	avocados
bean sprouts	bamboo shoots	bacon
beer	beef	breads
bittermelon	beef stock	broccoli
bok choy (white-stem cabbage)	cereals	brown and white rice
cabbage	cheeses	cantaloupe
Chinese cabbage	chicken stock	carrots
choy sum (flowering cabbage)	chili	cherries
cauliflower	chili sauce	chestnuts (unroasted)
celery	chips	chicken
cucumber	chocolate	Chinese peas
eggplant	clams	Chinese spinach
grapefruit	coffee	corn
green tea	crab	eggs
honeydew melon	deep-fried foods (w/oil)	fish (w/scales)
jasmine tea	duck	fresh ginger
lettuce	durian	garlic (cooked)
mushroom	goose	grapes
mung beans (green)	guava	green peppers (bell)
mustard cabbage	hot sauce	ham

YIN FOOD	YANG FOOD	NEUTRAL FOOD
oatmeal	ice cream	honey
ong choy (water spinach)	kim chee	kiwi fruit
oolong tea	lamb	lean chicken (w/o skin)
parsley	lobster	lean pork
pear	lychee	lean turkey
persimmon	lychee tea	lemon
squash	mango	long bean
turnip	milk	nuts (unroasted)
water chestnut	MSG	onions (cooked)
watercress	mustard sauce	oranges
watermelon	nectarines	oysters
wintermelon	peach	papayas
	pigeon	peanuts (unroasted)
	pineapple	pig's legs (and feet)
	pizza	poi
	plum	potatoes
	potato chips	prunes
	roasted foods	pumpkins
	red beans	seaweed (nori), unsalted
	scallops	snow peas
	shrimp	snow pea leaves
	squid	soy beans
	stir-fried foods (w/oil)	spinach
	toast	strawberries
	tobacco	tangerines
	yogurt	teas (black and brown)
		tofu
		taro
		tomatoes
		yams (sweet potatoes)

The above lists will help you in identifying the types of foods you most often consume. It will also help you in making better food choices. A sensible and desirable diet would be one which contains natural foods that are high in nutrients and fiber, low in fats, and contain a limited amount of seasonings like salt, soy sauce, sugar, hot spices, chicken or beef stock, and absolutely no MSG.

Here are a few of our families' kitchen cautions:

1. Stir-frying or deep-frying foods in oil changes the properties from Neutral or Yin to Yang and causes inflammatory diseases and high cholesterol. It is much better to steam, poach, broil, or stir-fry foods with water.

2. Green tea contains a lot of yin qualities. It can be used as a blood-thinner. Those who have low blood pressure should not drink it too often. Green tea is an herbal tea, and should only be taken when you are not feeling well, to clean the toxins from the body.

The Magic of Water

Water, nature's most generous gift, is valued by our bodies above all other nutrients. We can survive for weeks or months without food, but even a few days without water will result in certain death. Our bodies need at least eight (8-oz.) glasses of water each day to lubricate our joints, help in energy production, control our internal temperature, transport nutrients and waste, and assist in conducting chi through our systems.

In China, we say that water should always be consumed at room temperature or lukewarm. Warm water is less shocking in the lungs, and helps to wash down the mucus that might be clinging to the membranes that line the nose, mouth, and food canal (throat).

A couple of simple experiments will demonstrate why cold water and cold drinks are not good for your body. First, hold a glass of ice water in your hand for a minute or two. You will notice that your fingers will become numb. This is essentially what is happening in your system when you drink ice water. Second, mix a spoon of cooking oil or fat into a cold drink or ice water. You will notice that the liquid becomes lumpy as the fat hardens. According to Chinese herbal doctors, cold food and drinks slow down one's metabolism and weaken the digestive system.

Household Medicines

Both my father and grandfather were very famous herbal doctors in the districts in and surrounding Hong Kong. They always said, "Herbs have very good properties, but it is better to heal with fresh, nutritious food, and chi exercises."

I have followed their instructions with great success. The rule of thumb is: Chinese herbs (as well as other supplements) have good properties, but if used for a long period of time there are unpleasant side effects. I work under the premise that the body can produce natural healing to provide a counter-attack to sickness, illness, and ailment, if given the correct foods and exercises.

Listed below are common and readily available foods which have been used by the Chinese for medicinal purposes since ancient times.

Rock salt

Sore throat or mouth sores. Mix one teaspoon in warm water and gargle. 1/4 teaspoon mixed with warm water can be consumed before breakfast by those having high blood pressure. It should be stopped once pressure is down and back to normal.

Seaweed (laver, nori)

Promotes better blood circulation and helps those with low blood pressure. The high iodine content also helps to increase hair growth.

Spinach

Helps to regulate low blood pressure. It is high in iron.

Fresh ginger root

Relieves coughing. Also used to relieve stomach ache when one eats too much shellfish, crab, shrimp, lobster, and clams (Yang foods). Ginger helps to neutralize the high Yang energy which has built up in the body. Good also for motion sickness. Suck on sliced ginger root. Pig's legs and hard boiled egg, cooked in sweet vinegar, brown sugar, and ginger root, help a mother who has just given birth to hasten post-delivery recovery. It is often recommended by Chinese midwives. Ginger is the poor man's ginseng.

Dry lemon
Suck on a slice to dissolve mucus.

Raw garlic
Slice and rub on skin rash. It acts like an antiseptic.

Prunes and kiwi fruit
Prevents constipation.

Hot hard-boiled egg
Shelled and wrapped in soft cloth, gently roll on bruise on eye for ten to fifteen minutes.

Water chestnuts, Chinese parsley, and carrots
Boil equal parts of the water chestnuts, parsley, and sliced carrots in water for five to ten minutes to produce a drink that helps regulate high blood pressure.

Remember, our bodies need to have a balance of Yang (hot/male) and Yin (cold/female) energies. How often have you experienced, after consuming too much hot, spicy Yang-energy foods, a lack of sleep, or on the following morning a swollen throat, or swelling of the gums and tonsils? When this happens, the membranes in the nose and throat become sensitive to any dust, and you will start to sneeze or experience a running nose. Eventually, if you persist in this kind of diet, sinus problems and asthma develop. These conditions can be corrected by gargling with rock salt water. A small amount of this salt water may be swallowed to clean out the toxins. This should be followed by drinking herbal tea and eating Yin food.

Females should be careful about excessive consumption of Yin food to balance the Yang energy, as it may result in raising the level of potassium in the body, which can cause low blood pressure. Women going through their menstrual period should eat Neutral foods. Otherwise, their endocrine and immune systems will be affected, causing such problems as insomnia, nausea, and dizziness, or anemia (caused from the loss of blood).

Many of my students have come to me complaining of different ailments—constipation, back pain, insomnia, upset stomach, persistent cough. After asking them about their diets, I discovered that particular favorite foods imparting too much Yang or Yin were contributing to the cause of the problem.

One student ate raw garlic every day. He had trouble regaining his energy after a bout with the flu. His doctor said he had an overactive liver. I suggested he cook his garlic because raw garlic may be too strong for the walls of the internal organs, and should never be taken on an empty stomach. Soon his liver calmed, he was back to normal, and he said that—to his surprise—he actually preferred the flavor of cooked garlic, and the wonderful aroma it produced in the kitchen.

Another student was diagnosed with a fiber cyst in her abdomen. I asked about her diet and discovered she liked to chew on ice to combat the hot weather in Hawai'i. I always recommend no iced drinks and unchilled water because cold temperatures slow down the blood circulation.

Constipation plagued another student. He loved peanuts, roasted. I advised boiled peanuts instead. Soon his constipation was relieved. Another student with the same problem cut MSG (monosodium glutamate) from his diet and was also relieved.

Some of my students of Hispanic or Korean descent have tended to consume too many hot, spicy foods, which may cause depression and weight gain because of the high Yang energy. I have advised them that spices, salt, chili pepper and other hot ingredients result in swollen and inflamed glands, increase the appetite, deaden the senses so more and more spices are needed, cause dehydration, and compromise the kidneys. When they balance their diets with Yin and Neutral foods, their problems begin to dissipate.

For coughing I recommend two sources of relief. If you experience night coughing you have too much Yin (cold) energy. For this, drink tea made from ginger root, which balances the Yin with Yang (hot energy). Day coughing indicates too much Yang. To balance this, drink herbal tea. Too much herbal tea for females, however, may cause premature resumption of their menstruation.

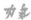

To me, the word "holistic" means total, complete, all-encompassing. I couldn't write a book about the healing properties of chi without including the dietary guidelines that were handed down from the Taoist monks to our family. We used to call this diet the "monk diet," but once we added all of the Western foods to the list, I changed the name to the Green Diet. It seemed to fit better. Green is the color of a rich landscape of growing things.

Now there are four things to balance: 1. the chi swirling through your external environment; 2. the chi you welcome into your body; 3. the chi your body generates; and now 4. the chi stored in the food you ingest. There is healing energy all around you. Take and balance what you need. It is not complicated.

Good luck, good health, and prosperity.

If You Heal One, You Heal the World

<hr>

Before I left Hong Kong and the tutelage of my father, I asked him a question that had been disturbing me for years. "I want to heal the world," I said. "There are so many people who have ailments that can be cured easily, but these people let things get out of control, and they eventually become diseased. Is it possible to help everybody? The world is so big."

Father was busy picking up the fallen leaves of a tangerine tree in the courtyard of his school. Without looking up, he said, "Bad apples, bad tree."

He knew that this type of explanation confused and frustrated me. He was testing my resolve. "What does that mean?" I asked.

He continued around the base of the tangerine tree. "When you look into someone's eyes, you can tell how healthy they are. The ailment or disease is only the fruit of the problem. The real difficulty lies in the 'tree,' the base of their physical body. That is where the origin of the affliction lies."

I felt like a puppy, following this bent old man in circles around the tree's trunk. "But what about healing the world?" I asked.

"You can only help one person at a time. When you heal one, you heal the world." He straightened, and looked me in the eye. "Bad apples, bad tree," he said. "This is true for an individual, a village, a city, a province, a country. It is all the same energy." He picked up his sack of leaves, and started walking toward the school. "When you heal one part of the whole, a change occurs. When you heal two parts, there is more change. When you heal three, a collective change begins to happen."

I followed close behind him, taking small steps and leaning forward to hear his words. Now I felt like a very old man, older than my father as we both shuffled toward the school. "You must affect change one person at a time. Don't worry about the whole. That will follow. Each part is important. Keep focused on what is in front of you." As he said this, he stopped, and I bumped into him. He turned to face me and laughed. "What did I say?" he asked. "Keep focused on what is in front of you."

I work with many different types of people; each is unique in their attitude toward life, physical ability, and ailments. And as I work with them, I remember, "You heal one, you heal the world."

When I started on this book project, people in my classes approached me and asked if they could tell their stories of how chi healed their illnesses. Here are some of their experiences:

My name is Ralph, but you can call me TURTLE.

Thirty years ago, while in the service, I suffered a severe nervous breakdown. Doctor after doctor examined me, but all they could give me was medication. The side-effects were terrible; uncontrolled shaking, delirium, and severe headaches. I knew there had to be a way to beat this illness, without medication.

After intermittent visits to mental hospitals for breakdown relapses, my family eventually gave up on me. They didn't know what to do. Neither did I. So, with my meds packed into a carry-on, I left home.

I heard that martial arts helped teach you to control your mind. So, I started looking for a class that might help me learn the discipline to fight my illness. A woman at my new job said that there was a man who taught martial arts in a local park every Sunday morning. So, that weekend I put on my sweats and walked to my destiny.

I expected to see people dressed in black martial arts outfits. Instead, there stood a group of normal looking people in shorts and tee-shirts talking to a handsome Chinese man and his wife. I had no idea that on that day I would find a remedy for this illness that had plagued me for years.

I've been training with Master Bond for over seven years now, and haven't had any nervous breakdowns. I don't take any medications either. My knees used to bother me when I tried to run or play tennis. Now there is no pain. I feel like Superman.

Master Bond is the one that gave me the name TURTLE. In chi kung, there is a posture called the "Golden Turtle." Master Bond promised me that if I perfected this stance, I would never have another breakdown. I worked so hard at it, and one day I showed Master Bond. He said, "Ralph, this posture is gold to you. For as long as you can do this, you will never have to worry about breakdowns. From now on, I'll call you TURTLE." I am so proud of that name.

I wish I could have learned this art at a younger age, because it opens your mind, opens your heart, and opens your spirit. I train every day, and I have a great teacher to guide me. These techniques have made me so happy, and I know I'll do this for the rest of my life. —Ralph

I'm 81 years old, and my friends call me a medical marvel. I've survived cancer and a massive heart attack.

About 2 years ago, I took a canoe trip up the Carrao River in Venezuela. Deep in the jungle, we came to a sharp bend. Water churned in turbulent swirls, and as our boat careened into the rapids, we capsized. Because of our remote location, help was very slow in coming. We bobbed in the strong currents for over an hour. While in the water, I almost passed out. My canoe-mates helped me hang on to the overturned boat until rescue came.

It took us five days to get home. When I got off the plane, my family took me to the hospital. I felt nauseated and dizzy, and my shoulder ached like a thousand knives piercing through my joint. At first, I thought it was just exhaustion from the canoe ordeal, but after an ECG, I was admitted for a ten-day hospital stay. The doctors said that the nausea, dizziness, and exhaustion was caused by a heart attack that I had experienced on my trip. I was also told that I needed tendon surgery on the rotator cuff of my left arm. I was a mess.

The doctors said that I didn't need a heart bypass, but that I had to take it easy and use a walking cane because my legs were weak and wobbly.

About a year and a half ago, I started taking Master Bond's chi healing classes. My health has steadily improved, and I do not need my cane anymore. The doctors say my heart is very strong, and although I was told that my shoulder would never regain its full range of motion, you could never tell by my tennis swing. There is no medical explanation for my current condition, that's why they call me a medical marvel.—Judy

My name is Miles, and I own a small business that I started seven years ago. The economy in our state is in a slump, and keeping the business going puts me under a lot of stress.

About a year ago, a family friend invited my wife and me to a free class on the healing powers of chi. I learned exercises that became tools to help me deal with stress, and within a couple of weeks I felt calmer and much more relaxed. I could effectively handle any situation associated with my job, conduct effective meetings, and make better decisions. Through this experience alone, I was sold on the benefits of chi therapy. But there were many more dividends to this healing practice.

I love to jog, but I frequently ran out of breath. It took me forever to recover from the run, and my muscles ached after every session. I blamed it all on aging. But after just a few weeks of chi therapy, my recovery time shortened, and the stretching exercises ameliorated any post-exercise muscular pain. I could exercise more frequently, and more effectively. I thought I'd found a gold mine of health.

Then, something happened that made me understand the copious power of chi energy. Four months ago, while driving through rush hour traffic, a truck rear-ended me in a four-car pileup. I was taking a large television set to the office, and had it propped behind the driver's seat. As the truck slammed into the back of my car, the television was thrown forward, driving its sharp corner through my chair, and into my back.

I'd never experienced back pain, so I was totally unprepared for this excruciating agony. I couldn't sit, stand, lie down, or walk without torturous pain. In situations like this, the last thing you want to do is stretch and exercise. The thought of chi exercise made me ache. My wife called Master Bond, and he came to our home. Gently, he coached me through a few movements. Almost immediately I felt my back loosen up. I did the exercises three times a day, and within a week all my pain was gone. It was like magic.

I've always been an avid exerciser, and to tell you the truth, when I first started doing the chi therapy, I thought, "This is much too simple to be effective." I was so wrong. As Master Bond says, "Simple and easy. That is the true beauty of this type of healing."—Miles

My name is Lillian, and I am 76 years old. I had taken t'ai chi ch'uan classes for 8 years, and enjoyed it very much. It made me feel good, but this form of t'ai chi never promised any healing benefits.

At that time, I had so many medical problems, there were seven doctors treating me at once. I had continuous respiratory distress like coughing, excessive mucus, wheezing, a voice that was hoarse, and a strange gurgling sensation in my lungs that made me suspicious of emphysema. I finally had to undergo lung surgery to treat a fungus growth and damaged tissue caused by 20 years of smoking.

My blood pressure and cholesterol were dangerously high, and since my family has a history of stokes and heart attack deaths, I was very concerned. And to top it all off, I contracted arthritis. My X-rays showed a combination of rheumatoid and osteo-arthritis. The throbbing pains at night kept me from sleeping. My swollen joints restricted my movements and my hand-grip was weak. Using medicated plaster on my painful joints seemed to temporarily relieve the pains in my hands and hips. I was coming apart at the seams.

A friend invited me to attend Master Bond's free class on the healing effects of chi. She said that the exercises were easy to learn, and very helpful in controlling her diabetes. So, two and a half years ago I walked into Master Bond's class with a body full of ailments, hoping to find some relief.

My friend was right, the exercises were so easy. But I had trouble with the dan tien breathing technique. I forced myself to practice every morning when I woke up, and every night before I went to bed. My only other option was to resign myself to my diseases, and succumb to their ravages.

Four weeks past, and I started to notice that the swelling and redness in my fingers and toe joints had improved. I remember waking up one morning, and my hips and my feet moved painlessly. Arthritis will always be with me, but the throbbing pains have subsided and I have the use of my hands and feet again. I can even swivel my hips.

After six weeks of diligent breathing exercises, magic happened! I was attending the chi class, and I became aware that my breathing was smooth, effortless. Now, I have one doctor, and my visits are like opening presents on my birthday. I used to go in for monthly blood pressure check-ups. One day, my doctor said that he wanted to see me every 3 months, then every 6 months. Today, with a small dose of medication, my blood pressure is normal again. I see my doctor once a year. Even my cholesterol count has improved.

I really can't believe the changes I've experienced in such a short time. The dan tien breathing technique and the exercises relieve stress and anxieties. They force me to relax. My lungs are clear, my stamina makes me feel like I'm 30 years old, and I've discovered that by practicing the healing chi exercise regimen, I am the healer. I have the power to effectively improve my own health. This knowledge lifts my spirits and calms my soul.

Master Bond reminds me all the time that my improved health is not a miracle. It's not miraculous. He says that I have effectively combined Western and Eastern medicine, and added a sprinkling of positive attitude, for successful "self-healing."—Lillian

Six years ago, I was overweight and was a possible candidate for a stroke or heart attack. For months, the paramedic that monitored my blood pressure nicknamed me his walking time bomb.

I'd been a martial arts student all my life. I worked out hard in my 20s and early 30s, but job schedules and personal dramas ate into my exercise time. Back then, t'ai chi and other martial arts kept me in shape. But when I turned 40, I gave up all forms of physical exercise. I unconsciously chose a very unhealthy lifestyle, increased my food consumption, and quickly gained weight. In a short period of a few years, I was 40 to 50 pounds overweight, and I'd started to build a very scary medical history of dangerously high blood pressure and cholesterol.

About a year ago, I met Master Bond and attended one of his free classes. That one-hour exercise session changed my life. Soon after, I got back into serious t'ai chi and chi kung training. Master Bond showed me exercises I'd never seen before. They were simple and easy, I could do them right away, no strenuous preparation training. My weight dropped, and so did my cholesterol and blood pressure levels. My body became more flexible, and one day I noticed that the stress-tension that I felt in my shoulders and neck had disappeared.

Last month, my younger brother (who is five years younger than I am) and I underwent a physical for our life insurance. It turned out that I was in the highest category for fitness, and he was in the category below me. This surprised everybody, the doctor, the insurance rep, my brother, and myself. I now have more strength and stamina than I've ever had.

This healing chi therapy has given me an intimate understanding of true internal strength. Master Bond's unique combination of dan tien breathing, chi exercises, and his emphasis on meditation cause the body and mind to unify and relax. This healing regimen builds muscular strength and vital stamina while promoting health, a sense of well-being, and youthful vigor. This would embarrass Master Bond (he is such a modest man), but he has truly saved my life.—Gregg

When I first started attending Master Bond's free chi therapy classes in January of 1997, I was on double doses of high blood pressure medication, taking 2 pills a day. Master Bond, my doctor, and I are so pleased with my progress. Now I'm down to 1 pill a day, and feeling fine.

A year ago, I was in a 3-car accident. A car slammed into me from behind, and pushed me into the car in front. The initial hit gave me whiplash, and when I smashed into the front car, I hit the steering wheel and bruised my ribs. To calm myself while waiting for the police, I did some deep, dan tien breathing.

The neck injury caused a suspicious tingling down my left arm, into my fingers. All that night, every chance I had, I did Master Bond's neck exercises.

The next morning, I visited my doctor. He ordered an ECG. I was fine. He asked me to rotate my head and arms in many different directions. To his surprise, and mine, there was no pain. The only pain I felt was from my bruised ribs. Master Bond told me to do dan tien breathing three times a day, and do some waist rotation exercises to let the chi into the painful areas. Within one week, the bruising was gone, and I haven't felt any discomfort since.

I've had other nagging ailments. I always had painful leg cramps, but after doing the exercises, they went away.

It is still amazing to me that such simple movements can cause such tremendous health gains.—Janet

I am 38 years old, and about to retire from the U.S. Army after 20 years of service. In 1996, I was diagnosed with arthritis and a degenerative joint disease in my right knee. My family has a history of arthritis, but the disease usually doesn't manifest itself until an advanced age. I have the dubious honor of being the youngest in my family to have ever contracted this disease.

Many doctors have told me that there is really no hope for a cure, and that I should deal with the fact that I will be in constant pain for the rest of my life. I was given Naproxen to take when the pain became unbearable. There are many side effects to Naproxen, and this medication really didn't help the pain much. Later, I started using Glucosamine Sulfate. It was very expensive, and didn't help either.

I've often heard that "when the student is ready, the teacher will appear." Well, it happened to me. A year ago, I started hearing about the benefits chi kung and t'ai chi. I decided to do some research. I checked the internet, and asked everyone I knew, including some Chinese people that worked on base. The outstanding endorsements impressed me.

One Friday, as I browsed the local newspaper's calendar section, I saw an announcement for Master Bond's healing chi therapy classes. It was like a door opened to me.

That Sunday, I went to class. I learned a lot of new techniques that promised to help me with my problem. I've been going every Sunday for about three months now, and I haven't had to go back to the doctor for more medication. I no longer wake up in agonizing pain, and the damp, cold rain doesn't bother me at all. The best part, though, is that I no longer take Glucosamine Sulfate. I don't need it. I don't hurt anymore.

About 6 months ago, I injured my back playing racquetball with my boss. I had trouble bending, reaching, and getting out of bed. Even laughing was painful. I took over-the-counter pain killers, but they didn't work. I was laid up for two weeks. Finally, I called Master Bond. He gave me a video tape he'd made, that provided specific exercises to release the blocked channels and meridians that were causing me pain. The exercises corrected the problem within a couple of days, and I've been doing them religiously ever since; 30 minutes each day, every day.

My back no longer gives me problems and I am playing racquetball again with my boss. In fact, I often leave him gasping for air.

I've also noticed that my breathing has improved, and I have much more energy and stamina. The chi exercises have given me back the power to run, bike, and play racquetball, things that I enjoyed before my knee and back injuries. My only regret is that I didn't start earlier.—Daniel

A little over two years ago, the epilepsy support group that I facilitate participated in a healing chi seminar given by Master Bond. I was so impressed with the simplicity of the exercises, I started attending Master Bond's classes.

Each week, I learned and perfected the movements. I practiced on my own every morning, and made gigantic strides in controlling my epileptic seizures.

The use of proper dan tien breathing techniques has enhanced every aspect of my life. Stress is one of the contributing factors to the onset of epileptic seizures, and since I began using the meditations and breathing, my feelings of stress have dramatically reduced. I feel more alive and mentally alert.

My seizure problems have lessened, and I know that this is due to the use and practice of the exercises and breathing techniques I learned from Master Bond.—Deborah

One day while in a local health food store, I had a conversation with a customer about breathing exercises.

She mentioned that every Sunday, a man named "Master Bond" taught the healing art of chi kung in a neighborhood park. She said, "The best part is that the class is free. Where are you going to get a better offer than that?"

I thought, what a beautiful and generous gesture. I was very anxious to participate, because I had been trying to teach myself chi kung movement using a book. I wasn't getting very far.

So, on a beautiful Sunday morning in January 1998, I took my first lesson. As we progressed through the movements, I got more and more excited. Master Bond's techniques and his dedication to teaching people to heal themselves using the healing chi was exactly what I was looking for.

I've been attending his classes, and practicing dan tien breathing and the chi exercises on a regular basis for about a year. The gains

I've made in stamina and muscle tone are wonderful. But the most surprising benefit has been my clarity of thought. I'm alert to things I never noticed before, and my memory has improved.

My brother is a karate master with 31 schools throughout the mainland United States. On his most recent visit, I invited him to one of Master Bond's classes. He was so impressed, he's decided to incorporate the dan tien breathing techniques and the chi exercises into his very successful martial arts programs.

This year I turned 58, and as a special birthday gift to myself, I decided to pursue an education in the healing art of acupuncture, and to master the self-healing powers of chi kung. It is such a blessing to know that through a combination of simple chi exercises and correct breathing, it's possible to achieve such a powerful physical, mental, and spiritual balance.—Gloria

My name is Barbara, and I'm 43 years old. About a year ago, a friend took me to Master Bond's chi kung breathing therapy class. I'd been looking for something new and healthy to add to my life, and was anxious to try something different. I'm a regular walker, and a strong believer in good health and taking care of my body, mind, and spirit. Chi kung has taught me the importance of correct deep breathing, and since I started taking Master Bond's classes, I've found that of all the healthy things I do, chi kung is most beneficial.

When I practice chi kung exercises, I have more energy. I know that I am giving my organs the blood and oxygen they need. Sometimes, when I'm stressed, and dealing with the pressures of everyday life threaten to overwhelm me, I stop, get quiet, and practice my deep breathing. I calm down immediately. It always makes me feel better.

The exercises are not difficult, and can be done anywhere, at any time. It is a program that fits easily into any lifestyle. At every class that Master Bond teaches, he shares the history and the method of using the breath. He also teaches us to visualize the oxygen as we send it down into our bodies, giving our organs the air and chi that helps keep them healthy and strong.

Thanks to him, I understand more and more how important breathing is. It's a personal choice. I plan to do chi kung for the rest of my life.—Barbara

Nearly two years ago, I was diagnosed with diabetes, and was given powerful medications to lower my glucose level. My friend Terry, who has diabetes, invited me to join Master Luk Chun Bond's healing chi exercise class. Terry had successfully controlled his diabetes through the exercises and breathing techniques taught by Master Bond.

It's been a year since my first class, and in February, when I had my routine physical exam, including blood tests, my glucose level was perfect. I was told that I could completely eliminate my medication because my glucose level had dropped considerably.

Three more physical examinations continued to show my glucose level as normal. I know that it was the chi kung exercises and a proper diet that helped to accomplish this amazing feat.

A couple of months ago, I started to play golf again. I feel so healthy and energetic. Golf is a hobby that I thoroughly enjoy. My high handicap has dropped, and I now participate in the Okinawa senior citizen tournament held once every two months.

When I decided to dedicate myself to learning and practicing dan tien breathing and the chi exercises, I received the greatest gift in the world: my life.—Tomiko

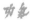

For years I have suffered with acid reflux, a condition where stomach acid, bile, and gas seem to get stuck in my throat. I've tried every antacid and home remedy. Nothing helps. If the problem occurs at night, I am unable to sleep, but if I do, I wake up vomiting.

In September, I started Master Bond's healing chi classes. I not only find I have more energy and flexibility, but wonder of wonders, I no longer have a problem with acid reflux. If I feel it coming on—

I do my chi kung exercises and the problem goes away.—Syndy

A lady never reveals her true age. I'll just say that I'm over 80 years old. After many years of practicing the 108 rhythmic movements of t'ai chi ch'uan, I joined Master Luk Chun Bond's healing chi classes. I enjoyed the exercise so much that I did the regimen twice a day.

In order to truly feel the power of this unique healing therapy, you must practice often. The rewards are a strong, healthy body, and a sharp mind. Both of these are highly valued by people of my age group.

Everything depends on the time and effort spent practicing. It has taught me perseverance, patience, and relaxation. After about 2 months, I was surprised to learn that I had lost 2 1/2 inches around my waist. The more I practiced, the more energetic and agile I felt.

It really doesn't matter how old you are, these exercises are easy, and can be done by anyone, of any age. Chi kung is an exercise of the body, mind, and of the spirit. The Chinese say that those who practice working with chi will be as graceful as a crane, gain the mystique of the dragon, the power of the tiger, the cunning of the mantis, the suppleness of the snake, and the wisdom of a sage. Learning these richly treasured, highly esteemed Chinese practices has changed my life. —Violet

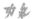

My name is Winfred, and I've been a student of Master Bond's for the past two years. I attend his class once a week, and practice the exercises and breathing every morning.

My wife and I usually arrive a few minutes early to take a quick walk before class starts. It's a good warm-up before beginning serious chi kung exercises.

Working with chi energy focuses the concentration of your mind and body, while teaching proper breathing techniques. When breathing properly, the body becomes fully charged with oxygen, thereby cleaning out the unwanted elements.

I have suffered from Parkinson's Disease for over 10 years. This is a degenerative illness which causes a loss of muscle control. The onset of the disease is gradual, with symptoms appearing minor at first, then progressing to uncontrollable shaking of the limbs, known as "tremors."

At times, these "tremors" inhibited my ability to hold things in my hands. My leg muscles would tighten, impairing my ability to walk, and because of this loss of muscle control, I am unable to stand for extended periods of time without swaying or shaking. I've spent many a sleepless night tossing and turning as bothersome tremors repeatedly shake me awake.

I once held black belts in Jujitsu and Karate, but this illness has made it impossible to engage in the rigors associated with the exercise and training required for these martial arts. I desperately needed to find a viable form of exercise that would provide some relief from my symptoms. I wanted something that would keep my body flexible and relax both my body and mind.

I tried a number of different exercise classes, but was not satisfied with the results. After more than a year of searching, my cousin Rose, a student of Master Bond's, explained some of the benefits of chi kung. She invited me to give it a try, and if it didn't help, I could always look for something else. After discussing the option with my wife, we decided to attend Master Bond's chi kung class together.

Three weeks after our first session, I began to feel like a different person. I was able to walk longer distances and stand for long periods of time without swaying or shaking. As time passed, I began jogging again, something that I'd previously given up because of the Parkinson's.

Learning Master Bond's chi kung exercises, combined with proper dan tien breathing, has truly been the best medicine for me. The exercises give me a good workout without being too strenuous, and provide me a way to energize mind and body. Through the breathing exercises, I've found a way to relax both my mind and my body, and am now able to fall asleep at night. Medically, my doctor can find no difference in my condition. I'm the one that has to live with this disease every minute of the day, and I know that Master Bond's techniques have helped me immensely. I am so happy, and tremendously grateful.—Winfred

I've always enjoyed excellent health. I haven't had a cold, the flu, or any common ailment in some time. About a year ago, I noticed that I was using the bathroom more often. I'd heard that frequent urination was a symptom of prostate cancer. So, I went to the health food store and bought some saw palmetto, zinc, and vitamins. I took them daily, thinking they would help keep this problem in check. When my fear became almost palpable, I went to see an internist. He told me that my PSA count was between 4 to 5, and that I shouldn't worry unless the count increased. In the last 12 months my PSA count jumped to 6.3.

My internist referred me to a urologist who insisted that I have a biopsy. In a straight-forward, rather cold manner, he made the point: one out of five cases is cancerous. I felt as though I was playing a game of Russian roulette, a pistol held to my head with a cancer bullet in one of the chambers.

I asked Master Bond if chi kung could help me. He was very encouraging, and he pointed out that chi kung exercises open certain channels to allow the life force to flow throughout your body. He showed me some exercises to do 3 times a day, then recommended specific foods to eat.

I followed his instructions religiously, and three weeks later, I met with Master Bond again. My urination problems had decreased, and I felt much stronger. Master Bond adjusted my exercise movements and corrected my breathing tempo (I was doing everything much too fast).

A week after Master Bond's adjustments to my chi kung technique, I slept through the night for the first time in a year. I went to bed, and didn't have to use the bathroom once all night. I was more energetic and enthusiastic. I really felt good. In fact, this was the best I'd felt in many years.

It is amazing what happens when you are ill. Things you take for granted, like sleeping soundly, waking refreshed, or even the ability to take a brisk walk, become distant dreams. And when you feel better, everything is new: colors are brighter, flowers are more fragrant, the sun more golden.

I finally did have a biopsy done. The test results were negative.

I'm breathing a sigh of relief, and have vowed to continue with these exercises. It's like putting money in the bank: my health bank.
—Richard

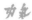

I am 69 years old, and have had Type II diabetes and a history of high blood pressure for nearly twenty years. At first, I had to take insulin shots. The oral medications were not adequately controlling my blood sugar level. I was informed by my doctor that I would most likely need to take insulin for the rest of my life. With such a prognosis, I decided to revamp my lifestyle, and take better care of myself.

The three most important elements for controlling diabetes are medication, exercise, and diet. With the help of my doctor, I mapped out a plan. I left the types of medications and dosages to my endocrinologist. As for my diet, initially I worked with a dietitian to help plan my meals. My wife was very helpful and willing to make whatever adjustments necessary to help me. I altered my diet drastically, and reduced or eliminated the intake of animal fat, sugar, sodium, and most dairy products. It took two years for this revised diet to become tolerable and surprisingly acceptable.

The exercise portion of my strategy included Master Bond's classes on the healing chi. I started attending his classes about two years ago, after watching a demonstration he'd done for our diabetes support group. Within three months I received the surprise of my life. After a routine examination, my doctor asked me if I would like to get off the insulin injections, and go back to oral medications. I, of course, was elated.

I truly believe that practicing Master Bond's healing chi and breathing power therapy played a significant role in controlling my blood sugar levels. I think Master Bond and his professional associates are doing an outstanding job of bringing happiness and good health to those seeking to restore or just maintain a sound mind and body.

Working with chi has become more and more popular. My doctor has seen its effect on my health, and many other physicians recognize chi exercises and dan tien breathing as precious sources of healing for many ailments. Doctors are wise not to reject this valuable restorative tool as a passing fad.

Within our chi class, a significant number of people have reported dramatic improvements in health. To me, it is neither a coincidence nor an accident that such positive, encouraging comments have come forward. Chi kung or breathing power therapy really works.—Terry

I am 27 years old, and I work as a Health Services Management Journeyman in the U.S. Air Force. I have suffered from lower back pain for over twelve years. I have been practicing with Master Bond now for almost three months and I have lost over ten pounds of weight, my energy is much higher, my appetite has improved, and I no longer go to sleep or wake up with lower back stiffness. In addition to lower back pain, I have also suffered from an acute fatty liver for over five years. My last blood test revealed that my liver enzymes were within a few points of the normal levels. I used to be hundreds of points above normal. I thank Master Bond for his unparalleled generosity in sharing this treasure of wisdom and healing called chi kung and t'ai chi. There truly is no price for this ancient art of healing and longevity. I'm looking forward to a long, healthy life! Master Bond, I am forever grateful.—Martin

I have practiced and studied t'ai chi ch'uan for many years. Recently, following a routine medical checkup, my doctor told me that my blood pressure was dangerously high. He suggested a change in diet, increased exercise, and medications with frightening names. I left his office, and embarked on a quest to find a holistic form of exercise that would help me heal myself without the use of medications.

A friend told me about a Chinese man who taught a free chi kung class once a week at a local park. Many of his students were impressed with their personal medical progress. My friend thought I might be interested.

My first meeting with Master Bond was very interesting. He gave me a video tape, and told me to do the exercises every day for a week, then come back and learn more in class. I progressed quickly through the recommended regimen, and soon joined his advanced class. I lost 10 pounds very rapidly, as though my body had been waiting for a way to rid itself of the excess weight. On the next visit to the doctor, the examination revealed a nearly normal blood pressure, still a little high, but with lower cholesterol levels.

I felt so good that I dropped my guard the following weeks, and slowly gained about half of the weight back. My blood pressure seems to have leveled off, though.

I have noticed that I experience some periods of completely normal blood pressure, especially after exercising and/or with medication. Although still under my doctor's guidance, I know that one day soon my blood pressure will be normal.

My stamina has definitely improved, and I've notice that the afternoon doldrums have disappeared. I can sustain longer periods of physical and mental activity, and as an unanticipated and rather dubious bonus, the practice of chi kung has revealed some "old wounds."

Master Bond says that when we begin to work with chi energy, we release blocks that have formed in our channels and meridians. Once these energetic pathways are opened, scars and old wounds are sometimes exposed. Mine started with lower back pain. I was in a car accident years ago, and I injured my back. I hadn't felt pain there in years. Master Bond helped me clear the scar, and the discomfort disappeared.

Just when I thought I could relax into the rhythm of good health, an old neck injury sustained while playing high school football started bothering me again. I had completely forgotten about this injury. It was as though my body, to prevent movements that caused pain, put a rigid, protective shield over the old wound. The exercises began to loosen the stiffness, and dissolve the shield to expose the painful, old injury. I persisted with the exercises, and now I have the youthful mobility in my neck I used to enjoy over 30 years ago.

Now I'm concentrating on healing an old wound in my ankle. I didn't realize what an active life I led as a youth. The old injury continues to show marked improvement, and to this date no other forgotten, heavily shielded "old wounds" have surfaced.

In chi kung, I have found a vehicle for self-healing. As I progress in my training, I continue to discover more and more about my body and mind. The exercises are an integral part of my life now, and I know that through the comprehensive practice of chi kung, as taught by Master Bond, I have found a pathway to optimum health.—Eugene

To all of my students and readers of this book: thank you. Now go and do your chi kung exercises, the first 16 secrets of chi.

Joy wei.

About the Author

Master Luk Chun Bond began his training at age six, learning from his father, a triple master. He shares his father's and grandfather's dream of teaching the true art of chi kung. He conducts private classes throughout Honolulu, and free weekly classes at Kapiolani Park.